CONTEMPORARY MANAGEMENT IN INTERNAL MEDICINE

JAY H. STEIN, MD, Editor-in-Chief

Professor and Chairman
The Dan F. Parman Distinguished Chair in Medicine
Department of Medicine
The University of Texas
Health Science Center at San Antonio
San Antonio, Texas

EDITORIAL BOARD

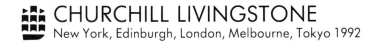 CHURCHILL LIVINGSTONE
New York, Edinburgh, London, Melbourne, Tokyo 1992

OBSTRUCTIVE LUNG DISEASE

STEPHEN G. JENKINSON, MD
Editor

Professor and Chief
Division of Pulmonary Diseases/Critical Care Medicine
The University of Texas
Health Science Center at San Antonio
San Antonio, Texas

CHURCHILL LIVINGSTONE
New York, Edinburgh, London, Melbourne, Tokyo 1992

ISSN: 1050-9607
ISBN 0-443-08872-1

The authors, editors, and publisher have exerted every effort to ensure that drug selection and dosage and descriptions of instruments and recommendations for their use set forth in all articles appearing in *Contemporary Management in Internal Medicine* are in accord with current recommendations and practice at the time of publication. However, many considerations necessitate caution in applying in practice any information appearing in *Contemporary Management in Internal Medicine*. The reader is advised to check package inserts for each drug for indications and dosages and the descriptions provided by instrument manufacturers for warnings and precautions.

Printed in the United States of America

Volume 2 Number 3
First published in 1992

CONTRIBUTING AUTHORS

Antonio Anzueto, MD
Assistant Instructor of Medicine
Division of Pulmonary Diseases/Critical Care Medicine
The University of Texas
Health Science Center at San Antonio
San Antonio, Texas

Charles L. Bryan, MD
Associate Professor of Medicine
Division of Pulmonary Diseases/Critical Care Medicine
The University of Texas
Health Science Center at San Antonio
San Antonio, Texas

William J. Gibbons, MD
Assistant Professor of Medicine and Physical Therapy
McGill University
Montreal, Quebec, Canada

Stephen G. Jenkinson, MD
Professor and Chief
Division of Pulmonary Diseases/Critical Care Medicine
The University of Texas
Health Science Center at San Antonio
San Antonio, Texas

Stephanie M. Levine, MD
Assistant Professor of Medicine
Division of Pulmonary Diseases/Critical Care Medicine
The University of Texas
Health Science Center at San Antonio
San Antonio, Texas

Jay I. Peters, MD
Associate Professor
Division of Pulmonary Diseases/Critical Care Medicine
The University of Texas
Health Science Center at San Antonio
San Antonio, Texas

Cynthia A. Zamora, MD
Assistant Professor of Medicine
Director, Pulmonary Function Laboratory and
  Respiratory Care Center
Division of Pulmonary Diseases/Critical Care Medicine
The University of Texas
Health Science Center at San Antonio
San Antonio, Texas

OBSTRUCTIVE LUNG DISEASE

CONTENTS

Volume 2   Number 3

OBSTRUCTIVE LUNG DISEASE

PREFACE

Obstructive lung disease is one of the leading causes of death in the United States, affecting millions of people. In this issue of *Contemporary Management in Internal Medicine*, the authors have strived to review both the means for proper diagnosis of obstructive lung disease and the modern approach to management of this large group of patients. Careful detail to pulmonary function evaluation at the first interaction with these patients can often narrow the diagnosis to an exact cause of the particular obstructive dysfunction. This may lead to very specific therapy, which might improve or at least halt the progression of airways obstruction. New breakthroughs in molecular biology have provided us with therapy for hereditary emphysema (α-1-antitrypsin deficiency), and the development of the technique of lung transplantation allows the possibility of definitive therapy, even in patients with end-stage obstructive dysfunction. As we are exposed to greater amounts of air pollution, patients with obstructive disorders of the lung will undoubtedly increase in number in the future. I believe the management presented in this issue will be very helpful in caring for these difficult patients and will serve to broaden our understanding of their obstructive pathophysiology.

Stephen G. Jenkinson, MD

PULMONARY FUNCTION INTERPRETATION IN PATIENTS WITH OBSTRUCTIVE LUNG DISEASE

STEPHEN G. JENKINSON, MD

Patients with obstructive lung disease are defined by very specific changes in their pulmonary function testing. Decreases in inspiratory or expiratory flow occur in these patients, causing either large or small airway obstruction. Pulmonary function testing is used both to diagnose obstructive lung dysfunction and to follow changes in airflow during the patient's course of treatment. Identifying the type of physiologic abnormality present by using pulmonary function testing can often narrow the list of causes of obstructive disease and allow one to determine accurately the degree of impairment present.

Abnormal values of pulmonary function tests are those outside the mean value obtained from a group of normal individuals matched according to age, height, and sex. These normal "predicted values" are calculated from specific prediction equations. The equations give a mean value for the group of normals and usually a range defined by confidence limits that include 95% of the variation of the normal group. Before a pulmonary function test is labeled abnormal, the results should fall outside the range in which 95% of people the same age, height, and sex would be found. All lung volumes obtained by spirometry or gas dilution studies must be corrected to body temperature saturated with water vapor (BTPS) in order to produce uniformity of interpretation from one pulmonary function laboratory to another.

Obstructive ventilatory diseases are manifested by a reduction of airflow through the conducting airways due to a decrease in their diameter or loss of their integrity. This condition has a variety of causes, including bronchial

To be labeled abnormal, pulmonary function test results should fall outside the range in which 95% of people the same age, height, and sex would be found.

The most common pulmonary function test used to measure airway obstruction is the forced expiratory spirogram.

smooth muscle contraction (asthma), airway collapse from loss of radical traction (emphysema), anatomic thickening of bronchial walls (chronic bronchitis), infiltration of the bronchial wall (tumor or granuloma), or aspiration of objects that mechanically obstruct bronchi (foreign bodies). Simple spirometry changes in patients with obstructive lung disease show enlargement of the total lung capacity (TLC) and increases in the residual volume (RV) (Fig. 1). The vital capacity (VC) may actually decrease depending on the amount RV increases. The most common pulmonary function test used to actually measure airway obstruction is the forced expiratory spirogram. This test assesses the rate of change in volume that occurs in the patients lung as a function of time.

The forced expiratory spirogram can be analyzed several ways to diagnose obstructive lung disease (Fig. 2). One of the simplest and most commonly used analyses is measurement of the forced expiratory volume exhaled after 1 second (FEV_1). A single value of this measurement can be compared with normal predicted values and different degrees of obstruction can be documented. The most widely used general classification for interpretation of obstructive lung dysfunction states that decreases in FEV_1 to less than 75% of predicted is mild obstruction, less than 60% of predicted is moderate obstruction, and less than 40% of predicted is severe obstruction. Measurement of $FEF_{0.2-1.2}$ (forced expiratory flow between 0.2 and 1.2 L of forced vital capacity [FVC]) and $FEF_{25\%-75\%}$ (forced expiratory flow, mid-expiratory phase) will also be abnormal in patients with obstructive airway disease. These measurements look

Spirometry

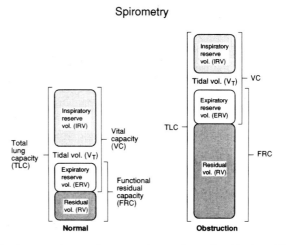

FIG. 1 Lung volumes in normal people and patients with obstructive lung disease.

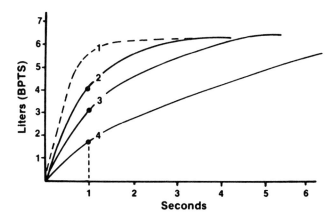

FIG. 2   The measurement of FEV_1 in a normal subject (1), a patient with mild airway obstruction (2), a patient with moderate airway obstruction (3), and a patient with severe airway obstruction (4).

at very specific portions of the forced expiratory spirogram. Neither of these two tests adds any more clinical information about an obstructed patient than the FEV_1 and both measurements are more variable.

FEV_1 measured as a percentage of the predicted value cannot be used to assess airway obstruction if a patient also has restrictive lung disease because all lung volumes are reduced. Since the FEV_1 is a volume, it, too, is reduced. A better way to evaluate obstruction in these patients is to measure the percentage of total FVC exhaled in the first second (FEV_1/FVC%). This measurement is called the *timed vital capacity*. A normal FEV_1/FVC% is 75%. (The ratio is age dependent and lower values may be normal in older patients.) This ratio remains normal even in the presence of severe restrictive lung disease or in patients with small airway disease. Measurement of FEV_1/FVC% is very useful at the bedside because it can be interpreted rapidly without having to consult a table of normal values. There is some decline of these ratios with increasing age, but even in the elderly the decline is very modest.

Mild obstruction is represented by an FEV_1/FVC% ratio between 75 and 60%. Moderate obstruction produces an FEV_1/FVC% ratio between 60 and 40%, and severe obstruction produces an FEV_1/FVC% ratio of less than 40%. When in evaluating the degree of obstruction in a single patient the FEV_1 measurement and the FEV_1/FVC% ratio are found to differ (e.g., FEV_1 equals 55% of predicted and FEV_1/FVC% ratio equals 64%), the FEV_1/FVC% ratio measurement should be used for the interpretation because FEV_1 can be decreased by concomitant restrictive disease. (The

FEV_1 measured as a percentage of predicted value cannot be used to assess airway obstruction in patients who also have restrictive lung disease, because all lung volumes are reduced in these patients.

Measurement of FEV_1/FVC% is very useful at the bedside because it can be interpreted rapidly, without consulting a table of normal values.

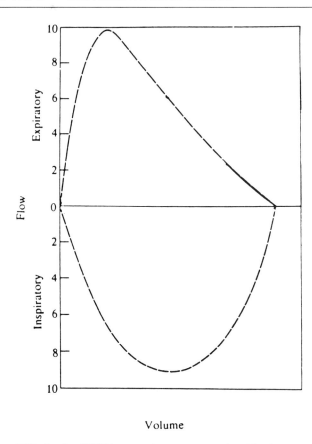

Volume

FIG. 3   An MEFV curve from a normal subject.

patient in this example would have *mild* obstructive ventilatory dysfunction.)

FEF can also be measured by plotting instantaneous airflow against lung volume during a maximum forced expiration. This is called a *maximum expiratory flow volume curve* (MEFV) (Fig. 3). The early portion of this maneuver is effort dependent and flow will increase in proportion to the intensity of effort. The latter portion is effort independent and flow depends on the resistance of the peripheral bronchi and the recoil pressure of the lung in the mid-vital capacity range. Computerized pulmonary function equipment is capable of extracting the FEV_1 and FVC from this curve and reporting them.

UPPER AIRWAY OBSTRUCTION

Patients with obstructing lesions of the upper airway can go unrecognized and misdiagnosed if pulmonary function testing is not closely examined. They have the same physiologic derangements as patients with asthma or chronic obstructive pulmonary disease (COPD), and often present with wheezing, shortness of breath, and severe hypoxemia. The type of upper airway obstruction in these patients can be either fixed or variable.[1] Fixed lesions do not allow the cross-sectional area of the airway to change regardless of the changes in transmural pressure. With variable lesions, however, the size of the airway can respond to changes in transmural pressure. Variable lesions are subclassified as intrathoracic or extrathoracic because of their location and response to changes in transmural pressure.[2] Pulmonary function testing can usually distinguish these various types of upper airway obstruction. It should be noted, however, that patients with bilateral obstruction of both main bronchi can have pulmonary function changes identical to patients with intrathoracic upper airway obstruction.

Pulmonary function tests used to diagnose and classify upper airway obstruction include spirometry and MEFV curves. In normal individuals, the maximum airflow achieved during the first 25% of a FVC maneuver is directly dependent on effort. With upper airway obstruction, flow at high lung volumes becomes limited much earlier by the obstruction and produces changes in the early portion of the forced expiratory spirogram. Rotman et al.[3] have defined variables that can be used to distinguish patients with upper airway obstruction from those with COPD or asthma. With spirometry alone, the $FEV_1/FEV_{0.5}$ (forced expiratory volume in 1 sec/forced expiratory volume in 0.5 sec) ratio in patients with upper airway obstruction is greater than or equal to 1.5. This is because $FEV_{0.5}$ is proportionately more reduced by obstruction of the upper airway since it occurs at higher lung volumes than FEV_1. This abnormality in the forced expiratory spirogram seen with upper airway obstruction has been referred to as "straightening" of the curve during the early portion of this test (Fig. 4).

Spirometry can sometimes be misleading in patients with variable extrathoracic obstruction. With this lesion, intraluminal pressure during expiration is much higher than extraluminal pressure. This actually causes the airway to dilate in the area of the obstruction during an expiratory maneuver.

MEFV curves are the pulmonary function tests of choice in diagnosing upper airway obstruction because they define the site of obstruction as well as document its presence. The various changes in MEFV curves from upper airway obstruction can be seen in Figure 5. With fixed obstruction, the plateau and limitation of flow is seen during both inspiration and expiration. Variable extrathoracic obstruction

Patients with bilateral obstruction of both main bronchi can have pulmonary function changes identical to those in patients with intrathoracic upper airway obstruction.

With spirometry alone, the $FEV_1/FEV_{0.5}$ ratio in patients with upper airway obstruction is 1.5 or greater.

MEFV curves are the pulmonary function tests of choice in diagnosing upper airway obstruction, because they define the site of obstruction as well as document its presence.

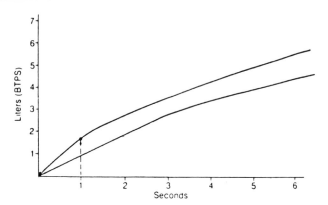

FIG. 4 Forced expiratory spirogram from a patient with asthma (top curve) and from a patient with upper airway obstruction (bottom curve). The patient with upper airway obstruction shows a "straightening" of the early portion of the forced expiratory spirogram.

produces flow limitation and a plateau only on inspiration for the reasons mentioned previously. Variable intrathoracic obstruction causes flow limitation and a plateau only on expiration because the pressure outside the lumen (pleural pressure) becomes much greater than the intraluminal pressure.

Patients with asthma usually exhibit increased airway resistance, a significant improvement in airflow in response to bronchodilators, and a normal DL$_{CO}$.

Although all patients with obstructive lung disease of any etiology have reduced flow rates on forced exhalation, the use of pulmonary function testing can sometimes be helpful in differentiating among the various causes of COPD. The different responses these patients show to selected pulmonary function tests are given in Table 1. Patients with asthma usually exhibit increased airway resistance, a significant improvement in airflow in response to bronchodilators, and a normal diffusing capacity of the

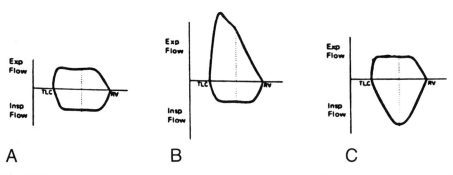

FIG. 5 MEFV curves from patients with (A) fixed obstruction, (B) variable extrathoracic obstruction, and (C) variable intrathoracic obstruction.

TABLE 1   Specific Pulmonary Function Patterns in Patients
           With COPD

	Asthma	Chronic Bronchitis	Emphysema
Decreased FEV_1	+ + + +	+ + + +	+ + + +
Decreased FEV_1/FVC ratio	+ + + +	+ + + +	+ + + +
Increased airway resistance	+ + + +	+ + + +	+
Decreased DL_{CO}	−	−	+ + + +
Response to bronchodilators	+ + + +	+	−

lung for carbon monoxide (DL_{CO}) because asthma causes reversible bronchial obstruction. Patients with chronic bronchitis also have an increased airway resistance and a normal DL_{CO}, but they usually have only a slight increase in flow after bronchodilators. Patients with emphysema exhibit little (if any) increase in airway resistance, no response to bronchodilators, and a marked decrease in DL_{CO} because emphysema is a disease of the terminal respiratory units characterized by loss of alveoli. A near-normal specific resistance associated with a decreased FEF is characteristic of emphysema, as airway resistance is measured in the absence of dynamic airway compression. The use of these pulmonary function tests combined with the clinical assessment of a patient can often reveal which cause of obstruction lung disease is most prevalent in a given subject.

Patients with emphysema exhibit little (if any) increase in airway resistance, no response to bronchodilators, and a marked decrease in DL_{CO}.

REVERSIBILITY OF OBSTRUCTION

When patients are found to have obstructive lung disease from causes other than upper airway obstruction, they should then be evaluated for their response to bronchodilators. If a patient improves after the use of a bronchodilator at the time of their pulmonary function testing, they are more likely to benefit from long-term administration of these drugs.[4] The interpretation of bronchodilator studies is often difficult because even small changes in reversibility of airway obstruction could be significant in a given patient if the obstruction is severe enough.

Studies in which bronchodilators were administered to normal persons have shown a mean increase in FEV_1 of 2.5% with a standard deviation (SD) of 3.9%.[2] If a positive response to bronchodilators is defined as a response of at least 2 SD above the mean response in normal individuals, then the FEV_1 must improve by at least 10% with bronchodilators to be considered significant. Other spirometric pa-

The interpretation of bronchodilator studies is often difficult because even small changes in reversibility of airway obstruction could be significant in a given patient if the obstruction is severe enough.

rameters, such as the FVC or $FEF_{25\%-75\%}$, have also been used by some to detect reversibility, but FEV_1 remains the best test for evaluating bronchodilator response. This is because increases in FEV_1, although not large, have a very small variability, which makes it a good discriminating test.[5] Some patients will not respond to a single inhalation from an aerosolized bronchodilator but may still have a reversible bronchospasm. These subjects may have used a bronchodilator prior to their arrival at the pulmonary function laboratory, or they may have an acute exacerbation of some other pulmonary disease that does not allow them to respond to the inhaled aerosols (such as bronchitis). Although their pulmonary function tests are interpreted as "no significant response to bronchodilators," the physician who ordered the tests may decide to administer bronchodilators for a period of days to weeks and then repeat pulmonary function tests to assess any "long-term" effects. Delayed improvement has been reported in some patients with "irreversible" airway obstruction after corticosteroid therapy.[6] There are no truly established criteria for a significant response in acutely ill patients because of the changes in severity of these patients' obstruction during an acute episode.

Delayed improvement after corticosteroid therapy has been reported in some patients with "irreversible" airway obstruction.

ABNORMAL GAS TRANSFER

A decrease in DL_{CO} is most commonly seen with emphysema, loss of parenchyma tissue from surgery, interstitial lung disease, and pulmonary vascular disease.

Measurement of diffusing capacity allows an evaluation of lung alveolar membranes and the pulmonary vascular bed. A reduction in diffusing capacity occurs with loss of alveolar surface area, thickening of alveolar membranes, loss of pulmonary capillary bed, increases in V/Q mismatch, or decreases in the amount of hemoglobin in the lung capillaries. Single-breath DL_{CO} is the most common measurement of diffusing capacity performed in pulmonary function laboratories, although a number of steady-state tests can also be performed. When the measurement of diffusing capacity is corrected for alveolar volume, it is referred to as the "specific" DL_{CO} (DL_{CO}/V_A). A decrease in DL_{CO} is most commonly seen with emphysema, loss of parenchymal tissue from surgery, interstitial lung disease, or pulmonary vascular disease. DL_{CO} should be less than 80% of predicted value to be considered abnormal because of the marked variability of the test.

Increased DL_{CO} can also occur and has been reported in patients with polycythemia, high-altitude dwellers, patients with intracardiac shunts, patients with congestive heart failure, and in some patients with asthma (thought to be caused by redistribution of perfusion). Increased DL_{CO} is normally seen during exercise because of an increase in blood flow into the lung with a resultant increase in blood-filled capillaries in the lung apexes. This same mechanism causes a slight increase in DL_{CO} when one assumes the supine position. All of the changes that cause an increase in DL_{CO} do so by increasing the amount of blood available in the pulmonary capillaries to take up carbon monoxide.

Increased DL_{CO} is normally seen during exercise because of an increase in blood flow into the lung with a resultant increase in blood-filled capillaries in the lung apexes.

INTERPRETATION OF PULMONARY FUNCTION TESTS

The information obtained from pulmonary function tests must be carefully assessed to avoid any misinterpretation. The manner in which a patient performs each test is extremely important in producing the results. Numbers generated summarizing pulmonary function tests can be misleading if the tests are not performed properly. The actual curves that produced these tests must also be examined in order to obtain a meaningful interpretation of pulmonary function data. Abnormalities like coughing, inconsistent effort, or mechanical malfunctions can easily be identified by direct examination of the pulmonary function tracings. Interpretations of lung function from a list of numbers produced by a computer without examination of the actual tracing should be avoided if an accurate assessment of a patient's pulmonary function status is to be made.

Abnormalities such as coughing, inconsistent effort, and mechanical malfunctions can easily be identified by direct examination of the pulmonary function tracings.

Other factors that can affect test interpretation include changes in function caused by variability in patients themselves.[7–9] A normal diurnal rhythm is now recognized that produces the worst function in the early morning, improves during the day, and again falls during the evening.[10,11] Large variations can also occur on a day-to-day basis in a single patient, especially if he or she has reversible obstructive airway disease. Patients may also inadvertently change their test results by doing such things as smoking immediately before the tests or using bronchodilator medications prior to arrival at the laboratory. This type of information must be made available to the person interpreting the pulmonary function tests before a patient can be labeled as abnormal or unresponsive to bronchodilators.

The pattern of worst function in the early morning, improvements during the day, and decreased function in the evening is now recognized as a normal diurnal rhythm.

Finally, an abnormal finding on a single pulmonary function test should always be confirmed at another time in order to avoid overinterpretation of the data and mislabeling of a normal person. Single determinations of bronchodilator studies should also be repeated serially before a patient with obstructive lung disease is denied the use of these drugs. The performance of pulmonary function tests require the interaction of a machine, a technician, a patient,

To avoid overinterpretation of data and the mislabeling of a normal person, an abnormal finding on a single pulmonary function test should always be confirmed at another time.

and the interpreter.[11] On a given day, problems pertaining to any of these four components can arise and produce data that do not truly represent a patient's baseline pulmonary status.

To avoid any problems with misinterpretation, the following rules should be applied:

(1) Pulmonary function equipment should be calibrated regularly.

(2) Volumes should be corrected for BTPS.

(3) Patients should be instructed not to smoke or use inhaled bronchodilators within 4 hours of testing, or use oral bronchodilators within 12 hours of testing.

4. Testing should be performed according to strict protocol.

(5) Repeat tests should be performed at the same time of day.

(6) Patient effort should be recorded as poor or good.

(7) Copies of pulmonary function tracings should be provided to the interpreter along with the computerized data printout sheets.

By following these simple steps, misinterpretation of pulmonary function testing can be minimized. Because of the psychological, financial, and legal implications of interpreting a patient's pulmonary function as being abnormal, any tests that are not clearly abnormal should be repeated before a final interpretation is made.

References

1. Acres JC, Kryger MH: Upper airway obstruction. Chest 80:207, 1981

2. Lazarus A: Pulmonary function tests in upper airway obstruction. Basics Resp Dis 8:1, 1980

3. Rotman HH, Liss HP, Weg JG: Diagnosis of upper airway obstruction by pulmonary function testing. Chest 68:796, 1975

4. Light RW: Use of the pulmonary function laboratory in the treatment of obstructive airway disease. Adv Asthma Allergy 5:10, 1978

5. Light RW, Conrad SA, George RB: The one best test for evaluating the effects of bronchodilator therapy. Chest 72:512, 1977

6. Scheinhorn DJ, Emory WB: Putting spirometry to use in your practice. J Resp Dis 2(8):8, 1981

7. Lapp NL, Amandus HE, Hall R, Morgan WKC: Lung volumes and flow rates in black and white subjects. Thorax 29:185, 1974

8. Wanner A: Interpretation of pulmonary function tests. p. 353. In Sackner MA (ed): Diagnostic techniques in pulmonary disease. Marcel Dekker, New York, 1980

9. McFadden ER Jr, Linden DA: A reduction in maximum mid-expiratory flow rate. A spirographic manifestation of small airway disease. Am J Med 52:725, 1972

10. Keogh BA, Crystal RG: Pulmonary function testing in interstitial pulmonary disease. Chest 78:856, 1980

11. Butler J: The pulmonary function test, cautious overinterpretation. Chest 79:498, 1981

PULMONARY REHABILITATION OF PATIENTS WITH CHRONIC OBSTRUCTIVE LUNG DISEASE

WILLIAM J. GIBBONS, MD

Clinicians have long recognized that morbidity from chronic lung disease has a significant cost, especially in terms of patient independence. Intolerable breathlessness is the proximate cause for limitation in ability to carry out normal activities.[1-3] Conventional therapeutic approaches, such as oxygen therapy and bronchodilator medications, are often not sufficient to ameliorate dyspnea and improve capacity to carry out activities of daily living. Accordingly, innovative approaches toward improving care of these patients while at the same time reducing its cost have been sought for many years. Pulmonary rehabilitation programs, which emphasize a multidisciplinary approach, patient education, and physical exercise training, have become increasingly popular as a means to supplement conventional treatment of patients disabled with chronic lung disease.

The purposes of this chapter are to outline the structure and functioning of these programs, to review the justifications for such programs, and to review and interpret the results of some components of this therapeutic intervention. This chapter will also cover certain new developments in clinical research that could likely impact on the conduct of pulmonary rehabilitation in the future. The reader is referred to several excellent reviews that have been published.[1,4-7]

Intolerable breathlessness is the proximate cause for limitation in ability to carry out normal activities.

Work supported by the Canadian Respiratory Health Network of Centres of Excellence.

PROGRAM STRUCTURE AND FUNCTIONING

The principle objectives of pulmonary rehabilitation are alleviation of the disabling symptoms, patient education, and return of the patient to independent functioning.

The American College of Chest Physicians and the American Thoracic Society have adopted a definition of pulmonary rehabilitation and provided guidelines for the conduct of pulmonary rehabilitation programs.[8] Patient selection, determining individual goals, and providing such therapeutic modalities as education, help with smoking cessation, psychosocial support, physical and occupational therapy, and exercise conditioning are all considered essential parts of such a program. The principal objectives are to alleviate disabling symptoms as much as possible, to educate the patients about their disease and treatments, and to return the patient to the highest possible level of independent functioning. As illustrated in Figure 1, pulmonary rehabilitation programs involve members from multiple health disciplines to realize these objectives. Although these members have separate functions to perform, each participates in the patient selection and evaluation process as well as in the education and treatment phases.

Pulmonary rehabilitation programs have been carried out in both inpatient and outpatient settings since the 1950s. One striking feature of pulmonary rehabilitation programs is the great variety one can find in terms of duration, patient population, therapeutic components, and other aspects. The reasons for such diversity probably lie in differences in local interest in such programs, available funding, and local biases regarding therapeutic components, among other reasons.

Patients with concurrent diseases that make exercise training risky or prevent them from attaining adequate exertional levels are usually not offered enrollment.

The patient selection and evaluation process attempts to include interested, highly motivated patients who complain of intolerable exertional dyspnea that interferes with

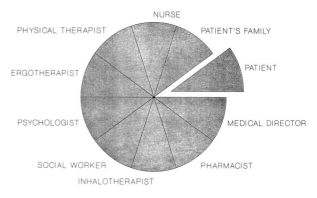

FIG. 1 Schematic diagram illustrating a multidisciplinary interaction during the operation of a pulmonary rehabilitation program.

their ability to carry out activities of daily living. Patients with concurrent diseases that might make exercise training somewhat risky or prevent the patient from attaining adequate exertional levels during exercise training are usually not offered enrollment. To this end all candidates undergo careful medical screening, including a history, physical examination, chest x-ray, electrocardiogram, complete blood count, biochemical profile, pulmonary function testing, and exercise testing. Examples of such concurrent problems include the presence of severe arthritis, severe peripheral vascular disease, severe exertional angina, and severe neuromuscular disease.

Traditionally, patients with chronic obstructive lung disease (COPD) have made up the majority of patients selected for participation in pulmonary rehabilitation programs.[4,5] These patients typically suffer from exertional breathlessness in the later stages of their disease and represent a large portion of all patients with chronic lung disease, making them an ideal group for pulmonary rehabilitation. Unfortunately, patients with very severe COPD, as indicated by very low FEV_1 (forced expiratory volume after 1 second) values and chronic carbon dioxide retention, have usually been excluded from programs because it was thought they could not benefit. However, recent retrospective studies have suggested that this subgroup of patients with COPD can experience the same degree of improvement in exercise capacity as less severely impaired patients with COPD.[9] In addition, patients with chronic lung diseases other than COPD can attain similar levels of improvement in exercise capacity after participation in a program.[10,11] These findings suggest that pulmonary rehabilitation can be regularly offered to many more patients than is the current practice in many programs.

Recent studies have suggested that this subgroup of patients with COPD can experience the same degree of improvement in exercise capacity as less severely impaired patients with COPD.

JUSTIFICATION FOR PULMONARY REHABILITATION PROGRAMS

Justification for the outlay of health care dollars to subsidize pulmonary rehabilitation programs remains controversial. It is common experience that pulmonary rehabilitation programs have individual patients who improve dramatically after participation, but no prospective, well-controlled study of large numbers of patients has been published yet to support pulmonary rehabilitation programs. Unfortunately, data used to document the benefits of pulmonary rehabilitation programs have often been retrospective and without adequate control groups. Nonetheless, data on the effects of pulmonary rehabilitation programs on utilization of health care resources, survival rate, pulmonary function, and quality of life are available.

The number of days of hospitalization per year and usage of other medical resources by patients who have received pulmonary rehabilitation decrease, suggesting significant savings in the cost of care in return for investment in pulmonary rehabilitation programs.[12-14] In one long-term study, this benefit was present up to 8 years after participation.[14]

It has been argued that long-term survival rates of patients with chronic lung disease are improved by participation in a pulmonary rehabilitation program, even when adjusting for level of pulmonary function (FEV_1) at the time of enrollment.[14] However, this assertion is based on comparison of survival rates with historical, rather than concurrent, untreated controls, which leaves the question unresolved.

Significant improvements in pulmonary function tests have generally not been found after participation in a rehabilitation program.[1,4,6] This is not surprising, given that the usual therapeutic components of pulmonary rehabilitation such as exercise training could not be expected to influence the fixed abnormalities in respiratory system mechanics found in patients with chronic lung disease. On the other hand, some investigators have claimed that the yearly decline in FEV_1 is slowed by participation in pulmonary rehabilitation.[14] Unfortunately, these data were compared against historical control data, but even if this were a true benefit of pulmonary rehabilitation its explanation is not clear. For example, smoking cessation alone could have been responsible.[15]

There is some question about what mechanism is responsible for the improvements in quality of life.

Most studies have shown improvements in quality of life after participation in pulmonary rehabilitation, as assessed either in an informal or formal manner.[14,16] There is some question about what mechanism is responsible for the improvements in quality of life. For example, could the increased medical attention given as part of a program by itself account for the improvement in quality of life, rather than the therapeutic components of a pulmonary rehabilitation program? The answer to this question awaits further research. Another important question about improvement in quality of life is, what is its duration after a participant finishes a program? In one well-controlled study, 11 of 24 (48%) of participants in a 2-week outpatient program continued to experience an improved quality of life 6 months after finishing the program.[16] This finding suggests that improvements are not permanent, and that periodic reinforcement is needed.

SELECTED THERAPEUTIC COMPONENTS OF PULMONARY REHABILITATION

Breathing Retraining

Breathing retraining is a technique commonly used today in pulmonary rehabilitation programs for patients with chronic respiratory diseases.[7,17–19] It is taught in the context of individual instruction with physiotherapists and also with group instruction at meetings such as "better breathing" clubs. The two most commonly used types of breathing retraining are diaphragmatic (or abdominal) breathing and pursed lips breathing.[18,19]

Although diaphragmatic breathing has long been known to respiratory clinicians, Barach[20] and Miller[21] were the first in the post-World War II era to vigorously promote its use in patients with respiratory disorders. Its goal is to reduce breathlessness and to improve the efficiency of breathing through slowing the respiratory rate and increasing the tidal volume.[17] Diaphragmatic breathing is supposed to accomplish this objective by assuring greater diaphragmatic participation during inspiration than that during unsupervised breathing. Initial reports in patients with chronic lung disease found that a rigorous program of diaphragmatic breathing yielded significant increases in diaphragmatic excursions, tidal volume, maximum breathing capacity, arterial oxygen saturation, and significant decreases in arterial carbon dioxide tensions over training periods of 6 weeks to 2 months.[22] Subsequent studies were performed to explain these salutary effects of diaphragmatic breathing by examining its effects on distribution of ventilation. No evidence of increased ventilation to the dependent portions of the lungs was found in patients with chronic lung disease,[23] whereas the opposite results were found in normal subjects.[24] Thus, the precise physiologic effects of diaphragmatic breathing remain unclear. Furthermore, physiologic confirmation of increased diaphragmatic activity during inspiration has been inconclusive in clinical studies of diaphragmatic breathing, making it difficult to determine whether patients actually performed effective diaphragmatic breathing. Although the use of a simple feedback method to facilitate learning of diaphragmatic breathing is attractive from a clinical standpoint, it can be potentially misleading. Outward displacement of the abdomen during inspiration is not necessarily always due to diaphragmatic contraction; it may also be due to the action of the abdominal wall muscles.[25]

A rigorous program of diaphragmatic breathing yielded significant increases in diaphragmatic excursions, tidal volume, maximum breathing capacity, arterial oxygen saturation, and significant decreases in arterial carbon dioxide tensions over training periods of 6 weeks to 2 months.

Dyspnea has been shown to correlate with activity of the sternocleidomastoid muscles during acute asthma attacks.

As part of the conventional diaphragmatic breathing technique, relaxation of the neck and chest wall muscles is usually encouraged to ameliorate breathlessness. Several lines of evidence support this practice. First of all, the diaphragm has a much lower concentration of muscle spindles and Golgi tendon organs than the intercostal muscles.[26] This finding suggests that the diaphragm may be relatively insensate compared to the intercostal muscles. Second, studies in humans have shown a relation between accessory muscle activity and breathlessness.[27,28] Changes in activation of the respiratory muscles were studied in normal subjects to determine whether they could account for changes in the sense of respiratory effort that accompany experimentally induced diaphragmatic fatigue.[27] Respiratory effort sensation correlated more closely with activation of the accessory muscles of inspiration than with diaphragmatic activation and fatigue.[27] Dyspnea has also been shown to correlate with activity of the sternocleidomastoid muscles during acute asthma attacks.[28] Taken together, all these lines of evidence suggest that therapeutic modalities that lessen the degree of accessory muscle activation can potentially result in less breathlessness. However, it is not clear what degree of intercostal muscle relaxation actually occurs during diaphragmatic breathing sessions. An objective measure such as electromyography to confirm reductions in intercostal muscle activity and provide feedback to the patient could represent a more effective method of ensuring derecruitment than simple verbal encouragement.

Pursed lips breathing is the other popular breathing retraining technique.[17–19] This technique teaches the patient to exhale more slowly by impeding airflow somewhat through pursed lips. One goal of pursed lips breathing is to lessen anxiety and dyspnea by level and pattern.[17] In terms of physiologic effects, although both minute ventilation and breathing frequency are reduced during pursed lips breathing, arterial carbon dioxide levels are not significantly altered.[29]

Whole Body Exercise Training

Whole body exercise training is a common component of most programs because it often results in an improved sense of well being, as well as an improved capacity to carry out activities of daily living. Exercise training may lessen exertional breathlessness by desensitizing patients to this uncomfortable sensation and by lowering ventilation requirements at any given level of exercise through an increased aerobic capacity (i.e., training effect) or through improved efficiency of exercise performance.[1] Commonly used whole body exercise training methods include walking, treadmill exercise, and bicycle ergometer exercise. Although an exhaustive review of pathophysiologic mechanisms of exercise limitation in patients with chronic lung disease is beyond the scope of this chapter, it is useful to discuss this topic briefly. Intolerable breathlessness, abnormal gas exchange and respiratory system mechanics, peripheral muscle deconditioning, and respiratory muscle dyscoordination and fatigue can all contribute to a limited maximum exercise capacity and exercise endurance in patients with severe chronic lung disease.[1-3] Medications such as corticosteroids may impair exertional capacity in these patients through the development of a peripheral myopathy.[30,31] Lastly, right heart dysfunction may also play a role in the exercise limitation of patients with chronic lung disease as suggested by the observation that maximal oxygen consumption correlates with right ventricular ejection fraction.[32]

Whether patients with severe chronic lung disease can perform sufficient exercise to achieve a training effect is controversial.[1] Belman and Kendregan found that certain aerobic enzymes were not increased in peripheral skeletal muscle of patients with COPD after 6 weeks of exercise training.[33] On the other hand, several studies have found elevated blood lactate concentrations at end-exercise in patients with COPD,[34-35] which are reduced after participation in a program of exercise training.[35] The exercise intensity or "target" needed to gain a training effect in patients with chronic lung disease remains controversial. The use of target heart rates, such as 60–90% of maximum,[36] may not always provide a training effect.[33] Some programs use target breathlessness levels instead.[1,4] Interestingly, a recent report suggests that a training effect can be obtained with very high intensity exercise training in these patients.[37]

Several controlled studies of exercise training using various protocols have documented significant improvements in exercise capacity compared to controls, with the beneficial effect lasting many months after finishing.[38-42] Typically, improvements in indices of submaximal exercise endurance such as 12-minute walking distance have been found; changes in maximum aerobic capacity have been inconsistent.[38-42] Improvement in 12-minute walking distance appears to be inversely proportional to initial 12-minute walking distance and directly proportional to FEV_1.[43]

The administration of supplemental oxygen to prevent significant falls in oxygen saturation during exercise is common practice.[7] In patients with COPD, supplemental oxy-

Exercise training may lessen exertional breathlessness by desensitizing patients to the sensation and lowering ventilation requirements at any given level of exercise through an increased aerobic capacity or improved efficiency of exercise performance.

Whether patients with severe chronic lung disease can perform sufficient exercise to achieve a training effect is controversial.

In patients with COPD, supplemental oxygen may lessen breathlessness through a reduction in ventilation at any given workload, thereby allowing the patient to exercise longer than without oxygen.

gen may also lessen breathlessness through a reduction in ventilation at any given workload, thereby allowing the patient to exercise longer than without oxygen.[44] One interesting observation about supplemental oxygen administration is that it permits longer endurance exercise even in patients who do not experience oxygen desaturation without it.[45,46] This effect presumably occurs through improvements in oxygen delivery to peripheral exercising muscle. Despite these interesting observations, oxygen is not commonly given to all patients undergoing exercise training, in part because of the financial cost of such a policy.

Ventilatory Muscle Training

Weakness can develop because of malnutrition, corticosteroid use, and other factors.

Ventilatory muscle training is another common component of most pulmonary rehabilitation programs.[4,6,7] The premise used to justify ventilatory muscle training is that inspiratory muscle dysfunction is prevalent among patients with COPD. Their inspiratory muscles are thought to operate at a mechanical disadvantage because of hyperinflation.[47] Weakness can also develop because of malnutrition,[48] corticosteroid use,[30,31] and other factors. Even evidence of inspiratory muscle fatigue has been reported in several studies of patients with severe COPD during vigorous exercise.[49,50]

Significant improvements in inspiratory muscle strength and dyspnea ratings have been documented with resistive breathing training when breathing strategy and pattern were carefully controlled.

Several methods have been used for inspiratory muscle training, including resistive breathing,[51,52] hyperventilation,[53] and inspiratory threshold pressure breathing.[54-56] The resistive breathing method involves inspiring through a device with variable small orifices that offer significant airflow resistance. This method primarily trains the inspiratory muscles for greater strength. Inconsistent results with resistive breathing training were reported in early studies.[6] These inconsistencies have been explained in part by variable training intensities being performed by subjects who changed their breathing strategy to minimize their inspiratory workload.[51] Another possible explanation is that some patients included for study did not have inspiratory muscle weakness to begin with, or had chronic inspiratory fatigue that would interfere with training. In any event, significant improvements in inspiratory muscle strength and dyspnea ratings have been documented with resistive breathing training when breathing strategy and pattern were carefully controlled.[51,52]

The hyperventilation method involves breathing at the highest flow rate consistent with the ability to maintain hyperpnea for 15 minutes (i.e., maximum sustainable ventilatory capacity).[53] This method primarily trains the inspiratory muscles for greater endurance, and has been effective in normal subjects.[53] In a study of patients with COPD, Levine et al. found increases in maximum sustainable ventilation, submaximal constant workrate exercise times, and maximum exercise capacity after 6 weeks of ventilatory endurance training.[57] Because this study involved a placebo, intermittent positive-pressure breathing, for comparison, these results are not conclusive regarding hyperventilation as an efficacious training method.[6,57]

The inspiratory threshold pressure breathing method involves inspiring against a consistent, reliable inspiratory load that must be overcome to allow inspiratory flow to occur.[54,55] This method trains for greater inspiratory muscle strength and endurance.[54,55] One advantage for the inspiratory threshold pressure breathing method is that it is not as affected by changes in breathing strategy and pattern as the resistive breathing method. It also offers the advantage of simpler equipment than that used with the hyperventilation method. Using inspiratory threshold pressure loads of 30% maximal inspiratory pressure, Larson et al. showed significant improvements in maximal inspiratory pressure and 12-minute walking distance in a well-controlled study of patients with chronic airflow obstruction.[54] In other studies, improvements in inspiratory muscle endurance in patients with COPD that were not due to changes in pulmonary mechanics have been reported.[55,56]

In a well-controlled study of patients with chronic airflow obstruction using inspiratory threshold pressure loads of 30% maximal inspiratory pressure, significant improvements in maximal inspiratory pressure and 12-minute walking distance were shown.

Exercise Training of the Upper Extremities

Clinicians have long recognized that breathlessness can be provoked by many types of activity in patients with moderate-to-severe COPD. In particular, breathlessness during upper extremities exertion is not uncommon in these patients.[58] Dyspnea in these patients is worse during exertion of the upper extremities compared to the lower extremities,[58] and worse when performing unsupported compared to supported upper extremities exercise.[25] Recently, investigations into the pathophysiology underlying dyspnea while using the upper extremities have been performed.[25,58,59] Simple arm elevation in patients with COPD results in an increased amplitude of sternocleidomastoid muscle electromyograph signal, increased end-inspiratory gastric and transdiaphragmatic pressures, and end-expiratory pleural and gastric pressures, suggesting recruitment of all of the respiratory muscles during this maneuver.[59] Dyssynchronous thoracoabdominal motion has been observed in association with the development of breathlessness during arm exercise in patients with moderate-to-severe COPD.[58] In a follow-up study using esophageal and gastric balloon catheters, Criner et al. showed that end-

These observations support the notion that upper extremities exercise provokes activation of all the respiratory muscles of patients with COPD, especially the accessory muscles.

inspiratory gastric and pleural pressures were more positive during unsupported arm exercise.[25] These observations support the notion that upper extremities exercise provokes activation of all the respiratory muscles of patients with COPD, especially the accessory muscles. The extra inspiratory burden for the accessory muscles while they are also performing important postural functions could lead to early fatigue of the upper extremities, resulting in a greater inspiratory burden for the diaphragm.[58]

Several approaches to ameliorating dyspnea during exertion of the upper extremities in patients with COPD have been tried. One approach has been upper extremities training programs for patients with COPD.[60–62] This approach is based on the premise that dyspnea during upper extremities exertion can be lessened by strengthening the muscles of the shoulder girdle and rib cage with exercise training. Breathlessness ratings and sense of well-being improved in patients with COPD in two studies of upper extremities training, but measurement of ventilatory muscle activation, strength, endurance, or recruitment patterns during upper extremities exercise were not performed in these studies.[61,62] Further studies using more appropriate controls and more sophisticated measurements should help better define the role of dynamic upper extremities exercise training in patients with chronic lung disease.

Another approach to ameliorating breathlessness in patients with COPD during exertion of the upper extremities has been arm bracing in the leaning forward position.[63] This maneuver is thought to provide mechanical support for the shoulder girdle and accessory muscles, thereby freeing the accessory muscles to better address their respiratory burdens. Support for this notion is provided by the observation that arm bracing has been observed to lessen dyspnea in many patients with COPD,[63] and that arm bracing increases the capacity for sustained hyperpnea in normals.[64]

Continuous Positive Airway Pressure

Patients with severe COPD develop dynamic hyperinflation during exercise,[65] presumably because expiratory time shortens and tidal volume increases during exercise in the setting of significant airways obstruction. Dynamic hyperinflation is detrimental to inspiratory muscle function during exercise because it shortens the operating length of the muscles,[47] increases lung elastance,[66] and increases the oxygen cost of breathing because of decreased efficiency of the inspiratory muscles.[67] It also presents an inspiratory elastic threshold load (i.e., intrinsic positive end-expiratory pressure, or "intrinsic PEEP"), to be overcome by the inspiratory muscles.[68]

The application of positive airway pressure has been proposed as a means to counterbalance the inspiratory threshold load offered by hyperinflation and oppose dynamic airway compression on expiration.[69,70] In studies on the effects of continuous positive airway pressure in patients with severe COPD during exercise, breathlessness ratings and exercise tolerance were found to be improved with the application of low levels (5 cmH$_2$O) of continuous positive airway pressure.[69,70] Unburdening of the inspiratory muscles by continuous positive airway pressure was postulated,[69,70] but investigation of the effects of continuous positive airway pressure on ventilatory muscle function was not performed in those studies.

In preliminary studies of patients with severe COPD during constant submaximal and graded workload exercise, inspiratory muscle activity as reflected by transdiaphragmatic and esophageal pressures was shown to fall with the application of modest levels (5 cmH$_2$O) of continuous positive airway pressure.[71,72] Dyspnea was ameliorated by continuous positive airway pressure in the majority of patients.[71,72] In a technically more sophisticated study, Petrof et al. administered continuous positive airway pressure levels of 7.5–10 cmH$_2$O to eight patients with severe COPD during constant, submaximal work rate bicycle exercise.[73] Esophageal and transdiaphragmatic pressure-time integrals fell, expiratory gastric pressure-time integrals rose, and end-expiratory lung volume did not change significantly with the application of continuous positive airway pressure during exercise. However, breathlessness ratings were not consistently decreased by the application of continuous positive airway pressure. These findings suggested that continuous positive airway pressure reduced diaphragmatic activity during exercise at the expense of the accessory inspiratory muscles (e.g., intercostal muscles).

The mechanisms by which the application of continuous positive airway pressure resulted in reduced inspiratory muscle activity in these clinical studies are probably complex. Applied positive airway pressure could have simply supplied part of the inflating pressure needed for inspiration, acted to counterbalance "intrinsic PEEP," and/or shifted some of the work of inspiration to the expiratory muscles.[73] Regardless of the exact mechanisms, these findings suggest positive airway pressure holds promise as an adjunct to exercise training of patients with COPD.

The application of positive airway pressure has been proposed as a means to counterbalance the inspiratory threshold load offered by hyperinflation and oppose dynamic airway compression on expiration.

Regardless of the exact mechanisms, these findings suggest positive airway pressure holds promise as a adjunct to exercise training of patients with COPD.

References

1. Belman MJ: Exercise in chronic obstructive pulmonary disease. Clin Chest Med 7:585, 1986

2. Gallagher CG: Exercise and chronic obstructive pulmonary disease. Med Clin North Am 74:619, 1990

3. Sue DY, Wasserman K: Exercise testing in the pulmonary patient. Curr Pulmonol 8:233, 1987

4. Ries AL: Position paper of the American Association of Cardiovascular and Pulmonary Rehabilitation: scientific basis of pulmonary rehabilitation. J Cardiopulmonary Rehabil 10:418, 1990

5. Hodgkin JE, Zorn EG, Connors GL (eds): Pulmonary rehabilitation: guidelines to success. Butterworth Publishers, Boston, 1984

6. Kelsen SG, Criner G: Rehabilitation of patients with COPD. p. 520. In Cherniak NS (ed): Chronic obstructive pulmonary disease. Chapter 56. WB Saunders, Philadelphia, 1991

7. Official statement of the American Thoracic Society: Standards for the diagnosis and care of patients with chronic obstructive pulmonary disease (COPD) and asthma. Am Rev Respir Dis 136:225, 1987

8. Official statement of the American Thoracic Society: Pulmonary rehabilitation. Am Rev Respir Dis 124:663, 1981

9. Foster S, Lopez D, Thomas HM: Pulmonary rehabilitation in COPD patients with elevated PCO_2. Am Rev Respir Dis 138:1519, 1988

10. Neiderman MS, Clemente PH, Fein AM, et al: Benefits of a multidisciplinary pulmonary rehabilitation program: improvements are independent of lung function. Chest 99:798, 1991

11. Foster S, Thomas HM: Pulmonary rehabilitation in lung disease other than chronic obstructive pulmonary disease. Am Rev Respir Dis 141:601, 1990

12. Hudson LD, Tyler ML, Petty TL: Hospitalization needs during an outpatient rehabilitation program for severe chronic airway obstruction. Chest 70:606, 1976

13. Sneider R, O'Malley JA, Kahn M: Trends in pulmonary rehabilitation: Eisenhower Medical Center, an 11-years' experience (1976–1987). J Cardiopulmonary Rehabil 11:453, 1988

14. Bebout DE, Hodgkin JE, Zorn G et al: Clinical and physiologic outcomes of a university-hospital pulmoanry rehabilitation program. Respir Care 28:1468, 1983

15. Fisher EB, Haire-Joshu, Morgan GD et al: State of the art: smoking and smoking cessation. Am Rev Respir Dis 142:702, 1990

16. Guyatt GH, Berman LB, Townsend M: Long-term outcome after respiratory rehabilitation. Can Med Assoc J 137:1089, 1987

17. Soria C, Walthall W, Price HL: Breathing and pulmonary hygiene techniques. p. 164. In Hodgkin JE, Zorn EG, Connors GL (eds): Pulmonary rehabilitation: guidelines to success. Butterworth Publishers, Boston, 1984

18. Rochester DF, Goldberg SK: Techniques of respiratory therapy. Am Rev Respir Dis 122:133, 1980

19. Falling LJ: Pulmonary rehabilitation-physical modalities. Clin Chest Med 7:599, 1986

20. Barach AL: Breathing exercises in pulmonary emphysema and allied chronic respiratory disease. Arch Phys Med Rehabil 36:379, 1955

21. Miller WF: Physical therapeutic measures in the treatment of chronic bronchopulmonary disorders: methods for breathing training. Am J Med 24:929, 1958

22. Miller WF: A physiologic evalaution of the effects of diaphragmatic breathing training in patients with chronic pulmonary emphysema. Am J Med 17:471, 1954

23. Sackner MA, Silva G, Banks JM et al: Distribution of diaphragmatic breathing during diaphragmatic breathing in obstructive lung disease. Am Rev Respir Dis 109:331, 1974

24. Roussos CS, Fixley M, Genest J et al: Voluntary factors influencing distribution of gas. Am Rev Respir Dis 116:457, 1977

25. Criner GJ, Celli BR: Effect of unsupported arm exercise on ventilatory muscle recruitment in patients with chronic airflow obstruction. Am Rev Respir Dis 138:856, 1988

26. Corda M, Von Euler C, Lennerstrand G: Proprioceptive innervation of the diaphragm. J Physiol (Lond) 178:161, 1965

27. Ward ME, Eidelman DE, Stubbing DG et al: Respiratory sensation and pattern of respiratory muscle activation during diapragmatic fatigue. J Appl Physiol 65:2181, 1988

28. McFadden ER Jr, Kiser R, de Groot WJ: Acute bronchial asthma: Relations between clinical and physiologic manisfestations. N Engl J Med 288:221, 1973

29. Mueller RE, Petty TL, Filley GF: Ventilation and arterial blood gas changes induced by pursed lips breathing. J Appl Physiol 28:784, 1970

30. Coomes EN: Corticosteroid myopathy. Ann Rheum Dis 24:465, 1965

31. Ferguson GT, Irvin CG, Cherniak RM: Effect of corticosteroids on diaphragmatic function and biochemistry in the rabbit. Am Rev Respir Dis 141:156, 1990

32. Morrison DA et al: Right ventricular dysfunction and the exercise limitation of chronic obstructive pulmonary disease. J Am Coll Cardiol 9:1219, 1987

33. Belman MJ, Kendregan BA: Exercise training fails to increase skeletal muscle enzymes in patients with chronic obstructive pulmonary disease. Am Rev Respir Dis 123:256, 1981

34. Sue DY, Wasserman K, Moricca RB, Casaburi R: Metabolic acidosis during exercise in patients with chronic obstructive pulmonary disease: use of the V-slope method for anaerobic threshold determination. Chest 94:931, 1988

35. Casaburi R, Patessio A, Ioli F et al: Reductions in exercise lactic acidosis and ventilation as a result of exercise training in patients with obstructive lung disease. Am Rev Respir Dis 143:9, 1991

36. Position stand of the American College of Sports Medicine: The recommened quantity and quality of exercise for developing and maintaining cardiorespiratory and muscular fitness in healthy adults. Med Sci Sports Exerc 22:265, 1990

37. Punzal A, Ries AL, Kaplan RM, Prewitt LM: Maximum intensity exercise training in patients with chronic obstructive pulmonary disease. Chest 100:618, 1991

38. Cockcroft AE, Saunders MJ, Berry G: Randomized controlled trial of rehabilitation in chronic respiratory disability. Thorax 36:200, 1981

39. McGavin CR, Gupta SP, Lloyd EL, McHardy GJR: Physical rehabilitation for the chronic bronchitic: results of a controlled trial of exercises in the home. Thorax 32:307, 1977

40. Booker HA: Exercise training and breathing control in patients with chronic airflow limitation. Physiotherapy 70:258, 1984

41. Sinclair DJM, Ingram CG: Controlled trial of supervised exercise training in chronic bronchitis. Br Med J 280:519, 1980

42. Busch AJ, McClements JD: Effects of a supervised home exercise program on patients with severe chronic obstructive pulmonary disease. Phys Ther 68:469, 1988

43. ZuWallack RL, Patel K, Reardon JZ et al: Predictors of improvement in the 12-minute walking distance following a six-week outpatient pulmonary rehabilitation program. Chest 99(4):805, 1991

44. Light RW, Mahutte CK, Stansbury DW et al: Relationship between improvement in exercise performance with supplemental oxygen and hypoxic ventilatory drive in patients with chronic airflow obstruction. Chest 95:751, 1989

45. Woodcock AA, Gross ER, Geddes DM: Oxygen relieves breathlessness in "pink puffers". Lancet 1:907, 1981

46. Zack MB, Palange AV: Oxygen supplemented exercise of ventilatory and nonventilatory muscles in pulmonary rehabilitation. Chest 88:669, 1985

47. Sharp JT: The respiratory muscles in chronic obstructive pulmonary disease. Am Rev Respir Dis 134:1089, 1986

48. Arora NS, Rochester DF: Respiratory muscle strength and maximum voluntary ventilation in undernourished patients. Am Rev Respir Dis 126:5, 1982

49. Grassino A, Gross D, Macklem PT et al: Inspiratory muscle fatigue as a factor limiting exercise. Bull Eur Physiopathol Respir 15:105, 1979

50. Bye PTP, Esau SA, Levy RD et al: Ventilatory muscle function during exercise in air and oxygen in patients with chronic airflow limitation. Am Rev Respir Dis 132:236, 1983

51. Belman MJ, Shadmehr R: Targeted resistive ventilatory muscle training in chronic obstructive pulmonary disease. J Appl Physiol 65:2726, 1988

52. Harver A, Mahler DA, Daubenspeck JA: Targeted inspiratory muscle training improves respiratory muscle function and reduces dyspnea in patients with chronic obstructive pulmonary disease. Ann Intern Med 111:117, 1989

53. Leith DE, Bradley M: Ventilatory muscle strength and endurance training. J Appl Physiol 41:508, 1976

54. Larson JL, Kim MJ, Sharp JT, Larson DA: Inspiratory muscle training with a pressure threshold breathing device in patients with chronic obstructive pulmonary disease. Am Rev Respir Dis 138:689, 1988

55. Goldstein R, De Rosie J, Long S et al: Applicability of a threshold loading device for inspiratory muscle testing and training in patients with COPD. Chest 96:564, 1989

56. Flynn MG, Barter CE, Nosworthy JC et al: Threshold pressure training, breathing pattern, and exercise performance in chronic airflow obstruction. Chest 95:535, 1989

57. Levine S, Weiser P, Gillen J: Evaluation of a ventilatory muscle endurance training program in the rehabilitation of patients with chronic obstructive pulmonary disease. Am Rev Respir Dis 133:400, 1986

58. Celli BR, Rassulo J, Make BJ: Dyssynchronous breathing during arm but not leg exercise in patients with chronic airflow obstruction. N Engl J Med 314:1485, 1986

59. Martinez FJ, Couser JI, Celli BR: Respiratory response to arm elevation in patients with chronic airflow obstruction. Am Rev Respir Dis 143:476, 1991

60. Ellis B, Ries AL: Upper extremity exercise training in pulmonary rehabilitation. J Cardiopulmonary Rehabil 11:227, 1991

61. Ries AL, Ellis B, Hawkins RW: Upper extremity exercise training in chronic obstructive pulmonary disease. Chest 93:688, 1988

62. Lake FR, Henderson K, Briffa T et al: Upper-limb and lower-limb exercise training in chronic airflow obstruction. Chest 97:1077, 1990

63. Sharp JT, Druz WS, Moisan T et al: Postural relief of dyspnea in severe chronic obstructive pulmonary disease. Am Rev Respir Dis 122:201, 1980

64. Banzett RB, Topulos GP, Leith DE, Nations CS: Bracing arms increases the capacity for sustained hyperpnea. Am Rev Respir Dis 138:106, 1988

65. Stubbing DG, Pengelly LD, Morse JLC, Jones NL: Pulmonary mechanics during exercise in subjects with chronic airflow limitation. J Appl Physiol 49:511, 1980

66. Pride NB, Macklem PT: Lung mechanics in disease. p. 685. In Meade J, Macklem PT (eds): Part 2, Chapter 37. Handbook of physiology—the respiratory system III. American Physiological Society, Bethesda, 1986

67. Levison H, Cherniak RM: Ventilatory cost of exercise in chronic obstructive pulmonary disease. J Appl Physiol 25:21, 1968

68. Tobin MJ, Lodato RF: PEEP, auto-PEEP, and waterfalls. Chest 96:449, 1989

69. O'Donnell DE, Sanii R, Giesbrecht G, Younes M: Effect of continuous positive airway pressure on respiratory sensation in patients with chronic obstructive pulmonary disease during submaximal exercise. Am Rev Respir Dis 138:1185, 1988

70. O'Donnel DE, Sanii R, Younes M: Improvement in exercise endurance in patients with chronic airflow limitation using continuous positive airway pressure. Am Rev Respir Dis 138:1510, 1988

71. Gibbons WJ, Marchini C, Garza C: Effect of continuous positive airway pressure on respiratory muscle function during exercise in patients with chronic obstructive lung disease. Chest 94:30S, 1988

72. Segarra J, Garza C, Gibbons W: Effect of continuous positive airway pressure (CPAP) on inspiratory muscle function during graded exercise in COPD. Am Rev Respir Dis 134:A91, 1989

73. Petrof B, Calderini E, Gottfried SB: Effect of CPAP on respiratory effort and dyspnea during exercise in severe COPD. J Appl Physiol 69:179, 1990

ASTHMA

JAY I. PETERS, MD

Asthma affects 5–10% of the population yet frequently remains undiagnosed or undertreated. Recent data suggest the prevalence and severity of asthma are increasing.[1,2] Despite our increased understanding of asthma and the improvement in therapy, there is evidence that the number of deaths attributed to asthma is also increasing.[3] The purpose of this chapter is to review the definition, natural history, pathophysiology, and therapy of asthma.

DEFINITION

The lack of a precise definition of asthma has been a major problem with studies of asthma. Clinicians would agree that conceptually asthma represents a disease characterized by bronchial hyperactivity, variable or episodic obstruction of airflow, and the presence of symptoms related to these pathophysiologic abnormalities.

More recent data suggest that the bronchial hyperreactivity relates to a chronic inflammatory disorder of the airways.[4] Bronchoalveolar lavage and bronchial biopsy of patients with even mild or subclinical asthma have demonstrated an increase in inflammatory cells, especially eosinophils. New technology has improved our understanding of the biochemistry, immunology, and physiology of asthma. Unfortunately, no single pathophysiologic defect or marker has been identified to more precisely define asthma.

A conceptual definition was proposed by the Committee on Diagnostic Standards of the American Thoracic Society:[5]

Bronchoalveolar lavage and bronchial biopsy of patients with even mild or subclinical asthma have demonstrated an increase in inflammatory cells.

> Asthma is a disease characterized by an increased responsiveness of the trachea and bronchi to various stimuli and manifested by a widespread narrowing of the airways that changes either spontaneously or as a result of therapy. The term "asthma" is not appropriate for bronchial narrowing which results solely from widespread bronchial infection, from destruction of the lung (e.g., pulmonary emphysema), or from cardiovascular disorders.

A committee of the American Thoracic Society[6] has defined reversibility as "a significant improvement in measurement(s) of airway obstruction greater than 1.65 times the coefficient of variation of the test(s) used to assess reversibility of the airways." Airway obstruction was described as the "presence of a significant obstructive ventilatory abnormality" in test of pulmonary mechanics with "associated periodic cough, tightness, wheezing, or dyspnea."

Such a conceptual definition still has many problems since it does not provide clear guidelines for distinguishing the patient with asthma from those patients with chronic obstructive pulmonary disease (COPD). Physicians tend to diagnose young, nonsmoking patients as "asthmatic" while labeling older, smoking patients as having "COPD." This definition is important since one should be more aggressive in utilizing anti-inflammatory pharmacotherapy with asthmatics.

Patients with COPD tend to have a slow, steady decline in forced vital capacity (70–90 ml/year) and diffusion capacity. Most patients with even chronic asthma and persisting airflow obstruction tend to maintain a normal diffusion capacity.

There are a number of features that can help to distinguish these two disorders. A clear history of paroxysmal respiratory episodes punctuated by return to normal function, a strong family history, or a lack of smoking and exposure to industrial irritants would suggest asthma. Blood or sputum eosinophilia, a high IgE level, and a very marked improvement in FEV_1 (forced expiratory volume after 1 second) with bronchodilators or steroids would also add support to the diagnosis of asthma. The laboratory response to bronchodilators cannot be relied on too heavily since some patients with COPD may have a significant response to bronchodilators. Patients with COPD tend to have a slow, steady decline in their forced vital capacity (70–90 ml/yr) and diffusion capacity. Most patients with even chronic asthma and persistent airflow obstruction tend to maintain a normal diffusion capacity.

PREVALENCE, INCIDENCE, AND NATURAL HISTORY

The lack of a precise definition has made it difficult to determine the incidence and prevalence of asthma. Depending on the definition between 7 and 20 million people have asthma in the United States.[7] The overall point prevalence of asthma (i.e., the prevalence of recently active asthma) in the United States is approximately 3–4%.[8–10] The cumulative prevalence (i.e., the prevalence of ever having had asthma) is 7% among males and 5–6% among females. Male predominance is most striking during childhood. Prevalence appears to be equal between males and females during adulthood.

The prevalence is relatively high in childhood, declines during adolescence, and rises again during middle ages.

The prevalence of asthma in the United States has increased by 33% in the last 20 years.[7]

The incidence of new cases of asthma also varies with age. In a population study in Michigan,[8] 50% of respondents dated the onset of asthma before the age of 10, while 25% experienced the onset of asthma after the age of 40.

The natural history of asthma has recently been reviewed by Weiss and Speizer.[11] They concluded that between 30% and 70% of children with asthma will significantly improve or have all symptoms of asthma resolve by early adulthood. Among childhood asthmatics, atropy and earlier onset of asthma is associated with increased severity. Asthma during adulthood is less likely to remit, although some adult asthmatics do experience remission or complete resolution of their disease. The frequency of asthmatic attacks has been found to be inversely related to the likelihood of remission. Approximately 60% of adult asthmatics who are symptom free will continue to demonstrate bronchial hyperactivity.

The mortality rate of asthma is difficult to assess since physicians often list the cause of death as respiratory failure or cardiopulmonary arrest. Recent U.S. mortality data indicate between 3,000 and 4,000 asthmatic deaths per year. Although this is equivalent to 1.5 deaths/100,000 person-years, it represents a doubling in asthma mortality over the past 20 years. Studies on asthma mortality indicate that 80–90% of deaths are preventable.[12] Most deaths from asthma occur outside the hospital or in an Emergency Department setting. The most common cause of death in outpatients as well as in hospitalized patients was found to be the inadequate assessment of the severity of airway obstruction by the patient or physician. The key to prevention of asthma mortality includes educating the patient as well as the physician. This concern has led the Division of Lung Diseases of the National Heart, Lung, and Blood Institute to develop through a concensus conference recommendations for the management of asthma in adults (Figs. 1–6).

The most common cause of death in outpatients and hospitalized patients in one study was inadequate assessment of the severity of airway obstruction.

PATHOGENESIS

Bronchial Hyperactivity

Bronchial hyperresponsiveness, an exaggerated bronchoconstrictor response to physical, chemical, or pharmacologic stimuli, is a key feature of asthma and correlates closely to the severity of asthma.[13] Bronchial hyperreactivity occurs in a unimodal distribution with the skewed portion of the curve reflecting hyperresponsiveness. Asthmatics fall at the most responsive end of the curve; however,

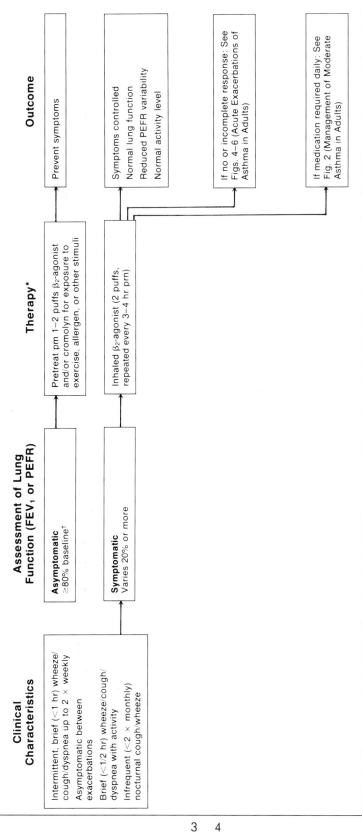

FIG. 1 Management of mild asthma in adults. *All therapy must include patient education about prevention (including environmental control where appropriate) as well as control of symptoms. †PEFR % baseline refers to the norm for the individual, established by the clinician. This may be % predicted of standardized norms or % patient's personal best.

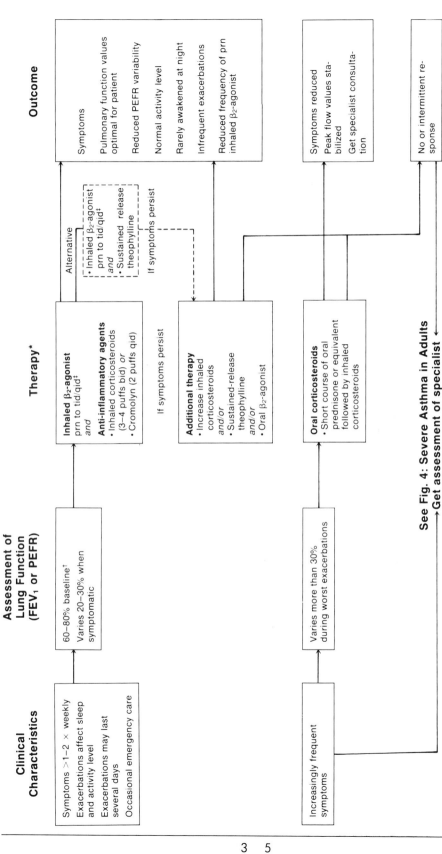

FIG. 2 Management of moderate asthma in adults. *All therapy must include patient education about prevention (including environmental control where appropriate) as well as control of symptoms. †PEFR % baseline refers to the norm for the individual, established by the clinician. This may be % predicted based on standardized norms or % patient's personal best. ‡If exceed 3–4 doses a day, additional therapy should be considered.

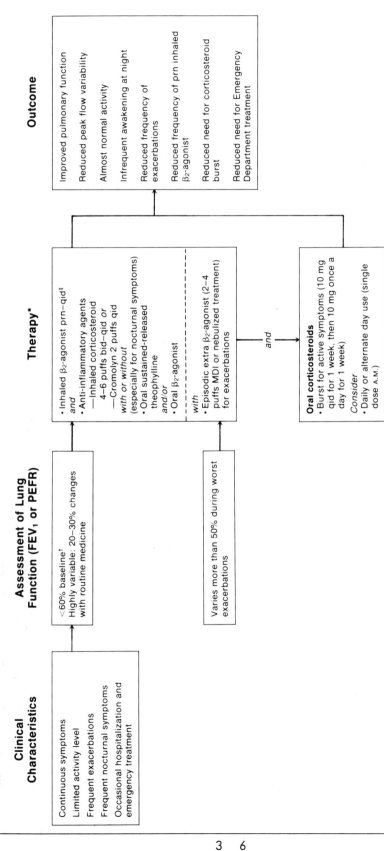

FIG. 3 Management of severe asthma in adults. *All therapy must include patient education about prevention (including environmental control where appropriate) as well as control of symptoms. Note: Individuals with severe asthma should be evaluated by an asthma specialist. †PEFR % baseline refers to the norm for the individual, established by the clinician. This may be % predicted of standardized norms or % patient's personal best. ‡If exceed 3–4 doses a day, additional therapy should be considered.

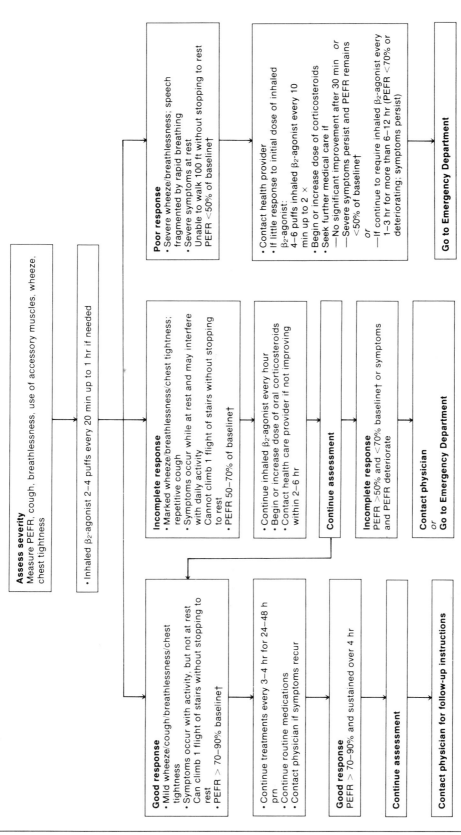

FIG. 4 Acute exacerbations of asthma in adults: home management.† PEFR % baseline refers to the norm for the individual, established by the clinician. This may be % predicted based on standardized norms or % patient's personal best.

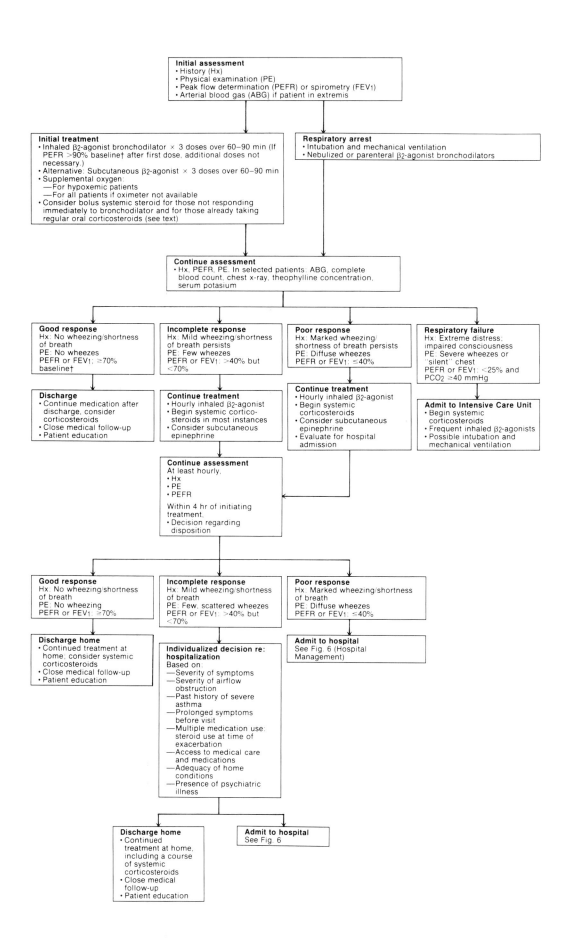

Initial assessment
- History (Hx)
- Physical examination (PE)
- Peak flow determination (PEFR) or spirometry (FEV₁)
- Arterial blood gas (ABG) if patient in extremis

Initial treatment
- Inhaled β₂-agonist bronchodilator × 3 doses over 60–90 min (If PEFR >90% baseline† after first dose, additional doses not necessary.)
- Alternative: Subcutaneous β₂-agonist × 3 doses over 60–90 min
- Supplemental oxygen:
  —For hypoxemic patients
  —For all patients if oximeter not available
- Consider bolus systemic steroid for those not responding immediately to bronchodilator and for those already taking regular oral corticosteroids (see text)

Respiratory arrest
- Intubation and mechanical ventilation
- Nebulized or parenteral β₂-agonist bronchodilators

Continue assessment
- Hx, PEFR, PE. In selected patients: ABG, complete blood count, chest x-ray, theophylline concentration, serum potasium

Good response
Hx: No wheezing/shortness of breath
PE: No wheezes
PEFR or FEV₁: ≥70% baseline†

Incomplete response
Hx: Mild wheezing/shortness of breath persists
PE: Few wheezes
PEFR or FEV₁: >40% but <70%

Poor response
Hx: Marked wheezing/ shortness of breath persists
PE: Diffuse wheezes
PEFR or FEV₁: ≤40%

Respiratory failure
Hx: Extreme distress; impaired consciousness
PE: Severe wheezes or ''silent'' chest
PEFR or FEV₁: <25% and PCO₂ ≥40 mmHg

Discharge
- Continue medication after discharge, consider corticosteroids
- Close medical follow-up
- Patient education

Continue treatment
- Hourly inhaled β₂-agonist
- Begin systemic corticosteroids in most instances
- Consider subcutaneous epinephrine

Continue treatment
- Hourly inhaled β₂-agonist
- Begin systemic corticosteroids
- Consider subcutaneous epinephrine
- Evaluate for hospital admission

Admit to Intensive Care Unit
- Begin systemic corticosteroids
- Frequent inhaled β₂-agonists
- Possible intubation and mechanical ventilation

Continue assessment
At least hourly,
- Hx
- PE
- PEFR

Within 4 hr of initiating treatment,
- Decision regarding disposition

Good response
Hx: No wheezing/shortness of breath
PE: No wheezing
PEFR or FEV₁: ≥70%

Incomplete response
Hx: Mild wheezing/shortness of breath
PE: Few, scattered wheezes
PEFR or FEV₁: >40% but <70%

Poor response
Hx: Marked wheezing/shortness of breath
PE: Diffuse wheezes
PEFR or FEV₁: ≤40%

Discharge home
- Continued treatment at home; consider systemic corticosteroids
- Close medical follow-up
- Patient education

Individualized decision re: hospitalization
Based on:
—Severity of symptoms
—Severity of airflow obstruction
—Past history of severe asthma
—Prolonged symptoms before visit
—Multiple medication use; steroid use at time of exacerbation
—Access to medical care and medications
—Adequacy of home conditions
—Presence of psychiatric illness

Admit to hospital
See Fig. 6 (Hospital Management)

Discharge home
- Continued treatment at home, including a course of systemic corticosteroids
- Close medical follow-up
- Patient education

Admit to hospital
See Fig. 6

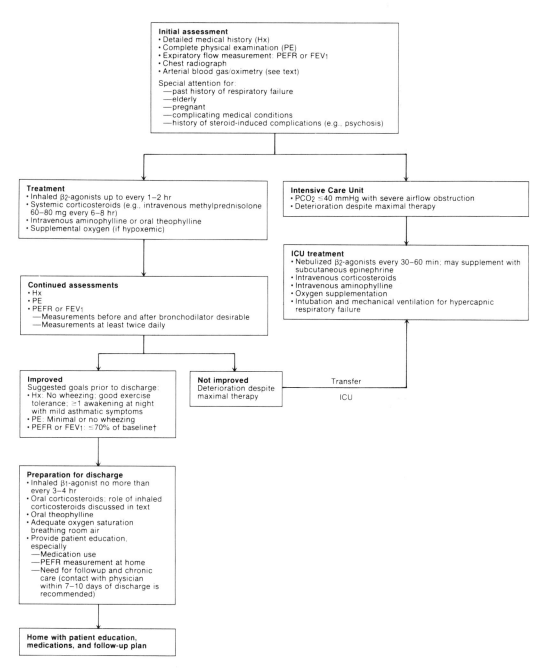

Initial assessment
- Detailed medical history (Hx)
- Complete physical examination (PE)
- Expiratory flow measurement: PEFR or FEV$_1$
- Chest radiograph
- Arterial blood gas/oximetry (see text)

Special attention for:
 —past history of respiratory failure
 —elderly
 —pregnant
 —complicating medical conditions
 —history of steroid-induced complications (e.g., psychosis)

Treatment
- Inhaled β$_2$-agonists up to every 1–2 hr
- Systemic corticosteroids (e.g., intravenous methylprednisolone 60–80 mg every 6–8 hr)
- Intravenous aminophylline or oral theophylline
- Supplemental oxygen (if hypoxemic)

Intensive Care Unit
- PCO$_2$ ≤40 mmHg with severe airflow obstruction
- Deterioration despite maximal therapy

ICU treatment
- Nebulized β$_2$-agonists every 30–60 min; may supplement with subcutaneous epinephrine
- Intravenous corticosteroids
- Intravenous aminophylline
- Oxygen supplementation
- Intubation and mechanical ventilation for hypercapnic respiratory failure

Continued assessments
- Hx
- PE
- PEFR or FEV$_1$
 —Measurements before and after bronchodilator desirable
 —Measurements at least twice daily

Improved
Suggested goals prior to discharge:
- Hx: No wheezing; good exercise tolerance; ≥1 awakening at night with mild asthmatic symptoms
- PE: Minimal or no wheezing
- PEFR or FEV$_1$: ≤70% of baseline†

Not improved
Deterioration despite maximal therapy

Transfer

ICU

Preparation for discharge
- Inhaled β$_1$-agonist no more than every 3–4 hr
- Oral corticosteroids; role of inhaled corticosteroids discussed in text
- Oral theophylline
- Adequate oxygen saturation breathing room air
- Provide patient education, especially
 —Medication use
 —PEFR measurement at home
 —Need for followup and chronic care (contact with physician within 7–10 days of discharge is recommended)

Home with patient education, medications, and follow-up plan

FIG. 6 Acute exacerbations of asthma in adults: hospital management. †PEFR % baseline refers to the norm for the individual, established by the clinician. This may be % of standardized norms or % patient's personal best.

FIG. 5 Acute exacerbations of asthma in adults*: Emergency Department management. *Therapies are often available in physician's office. However, most acutely severe exacerbations of asthma require a complete course of therapy in an Emergency Department. †PEFR % baseline refers to the norm for the individual, established by the clinician. This may be % of standardized norms or % patient's personal best.

some patients with chronic bronchitis or allergic rhinitis also demonstrate hyperreactivity. Increased bronchial responsiveness may also develop transiently in normal subjects after viral respiratory infections or after exposure to chemical irritants. Although there is some overlap between normals and asthmatics on bronchoprovocation studies, recent studies show these groups can be differentiate by dose–response curves. Woodcock[14] found that normal subjects reach a plateau with increasing doses of histamine (at about a 20% fall in FEV_1). Asthmatic patients not only required smaller doses of histamine (less than 8 mg/ml) but failed to reach a plateau at 60% fall in FEV_1. Bronchial challenge studies are rarely required to establish the diagnosis of asthma except in the setting of cough-variant asthma. It has been useful in screening employees who may require further protection and in documenting adverse effects in an occupational setting.

Much of the recent research in asthma has been directed at explaining bronchial hyperreactivity. There is compelling evidence in animal studies that the degree of bronchial reactivity is related to the extent of inflammation.[4] Increasing human evidence suggests that the increase in bronchial responsiveness seen in asthma relates to an inflammatory process in the airways.[15] There is considerable debate about which inflammatory cells and mediators lead to the histologic changes seen in asthma.

Structural Features of the Inflammatory Response

Although it has been recognized for over 30 years that fatal asthma is associated with marked inflammatory changes in the submucosa, recent studies demonstrate an inflammatory response even with very mild asthma.[16,17] The histologic features of asthma have been characterized by three findings: (1) an increased airway wall thickness caused by edema and an exudative inflammatory reaction, (2) smooth muscle hypertrophy and hyperplasia, and (3) mucus hypersecretion and hypertrophy. The theoretic concept states that an inflammatory reaction leads to tissue injury, resulting in exudation of fluid from the vascular space. This is followed by the appearance of platelets, leukocytes, and lymphocytes in the inflammatory site. Bronchoalveolar lavage confirms that albumin as well as inflammatory cells markedly increase in asthma.

The airway reacts to the inflammatory response like all other structures covered with a mucosal surface. First, there is shedding of mucosal epithelial cells. These cells sometimes coalesce to form clumps of cells called *Creola bodies*. Second, there is an increase in mucus from both the submucosal glands and the epithelial lining cells (i.e., the goblet cells). Pathologically, there is often a tenacious aggregate of cells, exudate, and mucus that plugs the airways in fatal cases of asthma. In asthma, there is also a reparative phase to the inflammatory response. Epithelial cells proliferate and cover the denuded surface. This rapid proliferation is associated with thickening of the basement membrane. Proliferation of the connective tissue and muscle leads to subepithelial fibrosis and thickening of the airway way.[18]

Inflammatory Cells

The inflammatory process appears to play a pivotal role in the pathologic changes in asthma. Additionally, inflammation of the airways with secondary release of mediators appear to be necessary for the persistent hyperreactivity that is characteristic of asthma. Airway inflammation results in epithelial damage with loss of cellular tight junctions. This loss of cellular integrity results in an increase in permeability of antigens and noxious stimulants, as well as exposure of the cholinergic irritant receptors that are located between cells. Therefore, recent research has focused on the inflammatory cells found in the airways and the mediators of the inflammatory response.

Mast Cells

For many years, mast cells were assumed to play the primary role in the pathogenesis of asthma since mast cells are marked increased within the walls of the airways of asthmatics. Histologic examination of patients who have died of asthma show marked degranulation of mast cells.[19] These cells are capable of binding IgE to their cell membrane, leading to the release of histamine, leukotriene C4, D4, and E4 (i.e., SRS-anaphylaxis [SRS-A]), prostaglandins, platelet activating factor, and factors that are chemotactic for eosinophils and neutrophils.[4] Recent data have shown that B_2 agonists, which are the most potent stabilizers of mast cells,[20] block the early response to allergens but fail to inhibit the late asthmatic response to allergens or to prevent bronchial hyperreactivity. Thus mast cells are involved in the immediate response to allergens but are unlikely to play a role in chronic asthma.

Eosinophils

Eosinophilic infiltration of the airways and peripheral eosinophils are characteristic features of asthma. Allergen in-

The inflammatory process appears to play a pivotal role in the pathologic changes in asthma. In addition, inflammation of the airways with secondary release of mediators appears to be necessary for the persistent hyperreactivity that is characteristic of asthma.

halation results in a significant increase in eosinophils in the bronchoalveolar lavage fluid at the time of the late asthmatic response.[21] The degree of eosinophilia in lavage fluid also closely correlates with the degree of bronchial reactivity.[22] Activated eosinophils have also been shown to result in epithelial damage by the release of major basic protein (MBP) from within the eosinophilic granule. Levels of MBP have been measured in asthmatic sputum at concentrations high enough to result in epithelial damage.[23] Eosinophils release a variety of other mediators, including platelet activating factor (PAF), leukotriene C_4, and oxygen radicals. The exact signal that brings eosinophils into the airway is not known. PAF appears to be the only mediator that selectively attracts eosinophils and is also effective in activating eosinophils.[24] Eosinophil production and migration are blocked by corticosteroids but are not effected by β agonists.

Alveolar Macrophages

Alveolar macrophages normally function as scavengers within the airway. Alveolar macrophages may be activated by antigens through activation of low-affinity IgE receptors present on their cell membrane.[25] Macrophages from patients with asthma release an increased amount of inflammatory mediators, including prostaglandins, PAF, and thromboxane.[26] Alveolar macrophages are also capable of releasing chemotactic factors for eosinophils and neutrophils. Unlike mast cells, macrophages fail to release their mediators when exposed to corticosteroids and are unaffected by β agonists.[4]

Lymphocytes

Animal studies demonstrate an accumulation of T-lymphocytes during the late asthmatic response to allergens.[27] These cells have also been shown to increase in the peripheral blood in patients with severe asthma and to decline with treatment.[4] Although little is known about the role of lymphocytes in human asthma, they act as immunomodulators and may play a role in chronic asthma. Methotrexate has been shown to ameliorate severe asthma, resulting in a reduction of corticosteroids needed to control the disease. Methotrexate reduces the proliferation and function of T-lymphocytes, which may suggest a role of T-lymphocytes in chronic asthma.

Mediators of Bronchial Hyperresponsiveness

The role of mediators and their effects on bronchospasm, chemotaxis, mucous production, microvascular leakage, and bronchial hyperresponsiveness has recently been reviewed.[28] Although a single mediator may have widespread effects on bronchial tone and inflammation, it is extremely unlikely that a single mediator accounts for the asthmatic response. For example, histamine causes many effects characteristic of asthma, yet does not cause bronchial hyperreactivity. Even potent antihistamines have not been shown to be clinically beneficial in the treatment of asthma.

Products of Arachidonic Acid

In humans, breakdown of phospholipid membranes to arachidonic acid leads to its metabolism into prostaglandins, thromboxanes, and the leukotrienes. Prostaglandin D_2 is released from human mast cells and is a potent bronchoconstrictor. The effects of prostaglandin D_2 are transient and its role in chronic asthma are unknown. Prostaglandin $F_{2\alpha}$ and prostaglandin I_2 (prostacyclin) are also produced in man and lead to bronchoconstriction. Prostacyclin is also a potent vasodilator and may contribute to inflammation and edema.

The sulfidopeptide leukotrienes, C_4, D_4, E_4, constitute the slow-reaching substance of anaphylaxis (i.e., SRS-A) and are potent constrictors of airways. They have also been shown to have an effect on microvascular permeability and mucociliary function.[4] Potent inhibitors of leukotrienes are currently being evaluated and may play a role in the future treatment of asthma.

The role of thromboxane A_2 in asthma has recently received increasing interest. This mediator is released by alveolar macrophages, neutrophils, epithelial cells, platelets, and fibroblasts. Specific thromboxane inhibitors have been developed and are undergoing clinical evaluation.

Platelet Activating Factor

Platelet activating factor (PAF) is the only mediator known to produce sustained bronchospasm. PAF is also derived from the membrane phospholipid of many inflammatory cells, including eosinophils, macrophages, and neutrophils. Inhaled PAF causes bronchoconstriction and bronchial hyperreactivity that has a peak effect at 3 days and may persist for 4 weeks.[29] In vitro, PAF is a potent chemoattractant of human eosinophils. Since PAF has a very short half-life, it probably acts as a trigger for other inflammatory events. Specific PAF antagonists, like ginkolide-B, may have a useful therapeutic effect in the prevention of eosinophilic inflammation.[30] Clinical trials will have to be conducted to evaluate the role of such drugs in chronic asthma.

Nervous System

The airways are innervated by the cholinergic, the adrenergic, and the nonadrenergic, noncholinergic (NANC) nervous system. The predominant tone of the airways is determined by the cholinergic tone maintained by vagal efferent activity. Nonmyelinated "C-fibers" lie beneath the tight junction of epithelial cells lining the airway and probably act as irritant receptors. Many stimuli such as sulfur dioxide, prostaglandins, bradykinin, and histamine stimulate these afferent receptors and may lead to bronchospasm through cholinergic mechanisms.[31] Anticholinergic therapy has been disappointing in the treatment of asthma; however, recent studies demonstrate three types of muscaric receptors in the cholinergic system.[32] Drugs such as atropine block the inhibitory prejunctional receptor (M_2 receptor) with equal affinity as the smooth muscle receptor (M_3 receptor). Development of drugs that selectively inhibit the muscarinic receptor on the smooth muscle (M_3) of airway may lead to reevaluation of the role of the cholinergic system in asthma.

β-adrenergic stimulation causes a dramatic reversal in bronchoconstriction. The possibility of an adrenergic abnormality has been extensively investigated and no consistent evidence exists for a primary defect in the β-receptor or in the function of this receptor in asthma. Adrenergic innervation of the airways is sparse and does not control airway muscle tone. All airway smooth muscle contains β_2-adrenergic receptors, which are affected by circulating catecholamines.

More recently, the trachea and bronchi have been shown to have innervation by the NANC nervous system. The role of the NANC nervous system in asthma is unknown but there is increasing evidence that neuropeptides may act as the neurotransmitters for NANC nerves.[4] It appears likely that this system has inhibitory nerves that release vasoactive intestinal peptide (VIP). One theory postulates that inflammatory cells release peptidases that lead to a deficiency of VIP in asthmatic airways. VIP may decrease the activity of the cholinergic nervous system and a deficiency could lead to increased bronchomotor tone.[33]

Another theory suggests an increase in activity of the NANC excitatory nerves. Animal studies suggest this system may function through the release of neuropeptides such as substance P or neurokinin A.[4] These tachykinins may cause bronchospasm, edema, and mucus hypersecretion. Since bronchial epithelial cells may play a role in breakdown of these substances, loss of epithelial integrity or function could increase the function of these neuropeptides. The role of the NANC nervous system awaits further study.

CLINICAL CONSIDERATIONS

Defining the Patient's Disease

The clinical history is important, not only in establishing the diagnosis of asthma, but in defining the precipitating event, or *trigger*. The clinical diagnosis is most often supported by a history of episodic dyspnea, cough, wheezing, or chest tightness. Exacerbations with upper respiratory infections, sinusitis, exercise, exposure to cold air, or emotional stress may be a prominent feature in some patients. Familial aggregation is well documented in patients with asthma and studies show a higher concordance among monozygotic twins compared to dizygotic twins.[11] A history of allergic rhinitis or atopic dermatitis is common in patients with allergic asthma and most asthmatic patients will give a history of nocturnal exacerbation of cough or wheeze when questioned specifically about nocturnal awakenings.

The pulmonary function laboratory may be helpful in documenting mild cases of asthma or those patients whose symptoms are believed to be of cardiovascular origin. Reduced expiratory flow rates that significantly improve after use of inhaled bronchodilators are seen in most asthmatic patients. Some patients develop chronic asthmatic bronchitis, which may be difficult to distinguish from COPD since both groups of patients have chronic obstruction often associated with air trapping (i.e., increased total lung capacity and residual volume). The chronic asthmatic patient should have a normal carbon monoxide diffusion capacity unless there is concomitant COPD, interstitial lung disease, or pulmonary vascular disease.

Some authors consider blood or sputum eosinophilia to be an invariable feature of asthma but documentation of this feature in controlled studies is lacking.

The initial evaluation of every asthmatic should include a search for factors that might precipitate or perpetuate the asthmatic attack (Table 1). An allergic component can be

Some authors consider blood or sputum eosinophilia to be an invariable feature of asthma, but documentation of this feature in controlled studies is lacking.

TABLE 1   Common Asthmatic Triggers

Respiratory infection: Respiratory syncytial virus (RSV), rhinovirus, influenza and parainfluenza, *Mycoplasma* pneumonia
Allergens: Animal danders, dust mites, airborne pollens
(grasses, trees, weeds), house dust, insect parts, fungal
spores, foods
Exercise
Environment: Cold air, ozone, sulfur dioxide, nitrogen dioxide
Emotions: Anxiety, fatigue, stress
Occupational stimuli: Animal handlers, antibiotic drug manufacturers, bakers (flour dust), woodworkers, spice and enzyme workers, plastic workers (anhydride), printers (gum ara-
bic), chemical workers (azo dyes, anthraquinone,
ethylenediamine, toluene diisocyanates), meat wrappers
(heated polyvinyl chloride), rubber workers (formaldehyde,
western red cedar, dimethylethanolamine)
Drugs: β-blockers, adenosine, propylene glycol (preservative
used in some asthma preparations)

demonstrated in 35–55% of asthmatic patients and may be
significantly higher in childhood asthma.[11] Many patients
are able to identify exposure to cats, house dust, feathers,
or other inhalants as a precipitating event of the asthmatic
attack.

When allergic asthmatics are given an inhalational challenge with an antigen to which they are sensitized, there is
an immediate asthmatic reaction in all subjects. This immediate response is characterized by a drop in pulmonary
function that reaches a nadir between 10 and 20 minutes
and reverses in 60–120 minutes without treatment.[4] Many
asthmatic subjects develop a late asthmatic reaction (LAR),
which begins approximately 4 hours after challenge and
reaches maximum intensity by 6 to 8 hours. The decline in
pulmonary function related to the LAR may persist for as
long as 24 hours. The immediate asthmatic response appears to be related to preformed mediators like histamine,
whereas the LAR is associated with an inflammatory response in the airways. Once subjects develop a LAR, they
demonstrate increased responsiveness to nonspecific stimulants like methacholine, histamine, or exercise for up to 6
weeks. Although the role of allergy remains controversial
in the etiology of asthma, evidence suggests it is an important factor in at least some asthmatics.

Upper respiratory tract infections frequently precipitate
or exacerbate asthma. Although the mechanism is not clear,
even normal individuals have been shown to have an increased bronchial reactivity to bronchial challenge during
an upper respiratory infection. The respiratory epithelium
may be damaged, exposing irritant receptors that could
cause bronchospasm if stimulated. Occult infection, partic-

ularly sinusitis, should be searched for in patients with recurrent or refractory asthma since appropriate treatment may significantly improve asthmatic symptoms.[34]

Aspirin sensitivity may be present in up to 25–30% of asthmatics. Symptoms may follow ingestion by several hours and patients may not associate the ingestion of aspirin with an exacerbation of their asthma. Although aspirin sensitivity may be more common in patients with nasal polyps, it is not restricted to this subgroup of asthmatics. Other nonsteroidal anti-inflammatory agents also induce asthma in these patients.

Other triggers include industrial inhalants. Occupational asthma has been estimated to account for 2% of all asthma and is a significant health problem.[35] Asthma may be produced by a prolonged exposure to industrial inhalants over months to years prior to the development of symptoms. Symptoms of occupational asthma are the typical asthmatic symptoms of cough, dyspnea, and wheeze. Initially, symptoms may be related to exposure to allergens or irritants at work and symptoms may resolve on weekends or vacations. Some occupational asthma progresses and may persist even after termination of exposure.[18]

Although classically asthma has been defined in terms of intrinsic asthma and extrinsic asthma, these distinctions are not useful clinically. Extrinsic asthma was believed to be caused by an allergen, to have seasonal variation in many patients, to occur in atopic individuals, and to manifest an elevated IgE level. Intrinsic asthma was believed to be perennial, and to occur in nonatopic individuals with a normal IgE level. Recent research suggests that all or most asthmatics have an inflammatory disorder of the lower airway and does not support the division of asthma into these two arbitrary classes. Overlap between these groups appears to be common and the division is not useful in predicting severity of asthma or in planning management strategies.

Clinical Patterns in Asthma

Clinically, asthma can present in variable patterns, from infrequent, mild, and episodic symptoms to perennial, intractable symptoms of status asthmaticus. Effective management requires an understanding of the patterns of asthma.

In one pattern of asthma, *cough variant asthma*, cough is the sole manifestation of the disease. The cough may be mild and intermittent or may be intractable and disrupt the patient's ability to sleep. Even in severe cases, routine pulmonary function tests may be completely normal. The

Aspirin sensitivity may be present in up to 25–30% of asthmatics. Because symptoms may follow ingestion by several hours, patients may not associate the ingestion of aspirin with an exacerbation of their asthma.

In "cough-variant asthma," cough is the sole manifestation of the disease. Even in severe cases, routine pulmonary function tests may be completely normal.

differential diagnosis includes sinusitis or rhinitis with postnasal drip, reflux esophagitis, or any inflammatory disorder involving the afferent nerves, which stimulate vagal efferent tone (otitis, pericarditis, pleuritis, gastroduodenitis). Patients with cough variant asthma have hyperreactive airways on methacholine bronchoprovocation and may require β-agonists, corticosteroids, or cromolyn to control their cough.

Exercise-induced asthma (EIA) is defined as a drop of 15–20% in baseline pulmonary functions with exertion. Most studies suggest that 70–90% of all asthmatics experience EIA.[36] During exercise, pulmonary function tends to increase over the first few minutes but declines after 6–8 minutes of vigorous exercise. After the return to baseline function, these patients enter a refractory period for up to 3 hours after exercise. During this period, repeat exertion at the same level of intensity produces either minimal or no change from baseline. The etiology of EIA is not known but a number of studies demonstrate a rise in plasma histamine and neutrophilic chemotactic factors in this disorder.[37] A small percentage of patients also form an LAR with EIA. Pretreatment several minutes prior to exercise with β-agonists or cromolyn controls the symptoms of EIA.

Nocturnal asthma refers to asthma that worsens during sleep. This appears to be a very common feature in most asthmatics but may be the predominant or sole symptomatic period in a subgroup of asthmatics. Individuals in this group are known as "morning dippers" because of significant dips in the peak flow early in the morning. Symptoms appear maximal between 2 and 4 A.M. and were initially believed to be associated with diurnal variations in cortisol and catecholamines. Recent data suggest nocturnal asthma may be multifactorial and that sinusitis, gastroesophageal reflux, and environmental allergies may play a significant role in this disorder.[38]

Chronic asthma describes a class of asthma in which symptoms are persistent to some degree throughout the year. The National Institute of Health's "Expert Panel on the Management of Asthma" divided chronic asthma into mild, moderate, and severe (see Figs. 1–3). *Mild asthma* was defined as asthma that occurred up to 2 times per week and lasted for less than 1 hour at rest or ½ hour after activity and when patients had nocturnal symptoms less than 2 times per month. *Moderate asthma* was defined as asthma that occurred more frequently than 1 or 2 times per week or when exacerbations affected sleep or the level of activity. Exacerbations in this group may last for several days. *Severe asthma* by definition included asthmatic patients with continuous symptoms and limited activity level. Frequent exacerbations and nocturnal symptoms are characteristic of this group. The algorithms created for each group of asthmatics (see Figs. 1–3) should act only as a guide since each patient's therapy should be individualized.

TREATMENT

The goal of asthma therapy is to prevent the symptoms of asthma and normalize activity back to the patient's baseline. When asthma exacerbates, the goal shifts to avoidance of hospitalization by early intensification of therapy. Sometimes this goal is not possible and the clinician must direct therapy toward prevention of respiratory failure and mortality associated with severe asthma. Toward these goals, every physician should make an effort to decrease the patient's airway hyperreactivity and attempt to prevent it from increasing. The increased awareness that inflammation plays a primary role in airway hyperreactivity and in exacerbation of asthma suggests a primary role for medications that reduce this inflammation process. Since the level of hyperactivity changes over time, newer recommendations in therapy begin with patient education and the teaching of patient self-management skills.

The mainstay of asthma therapy is pharmacologic agents which either control patient's symptoms or act to prevent exacerbations. In patients with known allergic triggers for their asthma, simple avoidance of the allergen has been shown to improve symptoms, lead to reductions in medication, and reduce bronchial hyperreactivity.[39] The role of immunotherapy in asthma is controversial but recent evidence suggests there may be a role of immunotherapy in patients whose asthma is poorly controlled despite avoidance of the allergen and pharmacotherapy. This topic is beyond the scope of this chapter but has been reviewed recently.[40]

β-adrenergic Agents

β_2-agonists are the most potent drugs currently available to acutely control the symptoms of asthma. These drugs lead to rapid bronchodilatation (within minutes) that lasts for 4–8 hours; however, their ability to prevent bronchoconstriction is of shorter duration (Table 2). This class of drug stimulates the β_2-adrenergic receptor, which activates adenyl cyclase. Adenyl cyclase produces an increase in cyclic AMP within the cell and results in smooth muscle relaxation, skeletal muscle stimulation, and mast cell stabilization.[4] β_2-agonist activation also stimulates gluconeogenesis

TABLE 2 Selectivity, Potency, and Duration of Action of the β-Adrenergic Agonists

Agent	Selectivity			Duration of Action		
	β_1	β_2	β_2 Potency*	Bronchodilation (hrs)	Protection (hrs)†	Oral Formulation
Isoproterenol	+ + + +	+ + + +	1	0.5–2	0.5–1.0	No
Isotharine	+ +	+ + +	6	0.5–2	0.5–1.0	No
Metaproterenol	+ + +	+ + +	15	3–4	1–2	Yes
Albuterol	+	+ + + +	2	4–8	2–4	Yes
Terbutaline	+	– – –	4	4–8	2–4	Yes
Bitolterol	+	+ + +	5	4–8	2–4	No
Pirbuterol	+	+ + + +	5	4–8	2–4	No
Formoterol	+	+ + + +	0.24	8–12	8–12	No
Salmeterol	+	+ + + +	0.50	8–12	—	No

* Relative molar potency: 1 = most potent.
† Refers to the duraton of time that bronchoconstriction may be prevented.

and insulin release, which produces a intercellular shift in serum potassium and may result in mild to moderate hypokalemia. β_2-Agonists also produce vascular smooth muscle relaxation, which results in vasodilatation and reflex tachycardia. There is also evidence of direct stimulation of cardiac β_2-adrenergic receptors, resulting in a positive chronotropic response, as well as some β_1-receptor stimulation with high concentrations of β_2-agonist.[4]

Nonselective β-agonists stimulate the β_1-receptor, which results in excessive cardiac stimulation and may produce arrythmias or myocardial ischemia. There is no rationale for using nonselective β-agonists in the treatment of asthma. Table 2 compares the β-adrenergic agonists available for the treatment of asthma. Longer-acting β_2-agonists (formoterol and salmeterol) are currently undergoing clinical trials. Salmeterol may be effective for more than 12 hours and may prove useful in controlling nocturnal asthma.

β_2-agonists relax smooth muscle regardless of the mechanism of bronchoconstriction. This feature has established them as the bronchodilators of choice in the treatment of asthma. When administered in equipotent doses, all of these drugs will produce an equal amount of bronchial relaxation; the only differences will be in the duration of action and the potential side effects. Clinical studies have shown that the dose–response relationship and the duration of activity are affected by the level of bronchoconstriction.[41] This has led to the understanding that severe exacerbations of asthma require more frequent and higher doses of β-agonist than routinely prescribed. The ability to increase the dose 5–10 times the dose used in chronic stable asthma contributes to the efficacy in reversing the bronchospasm of severe asthma.

The only disadvantage of inhaled β-agonists is the short duration of action and the difficulty some patients have in

Beta-2 agonists relax smooth muscle regardless of the mechanism of bronchoconstriction. This feature has established them as the bronchodilator of choice in the treatment of asthma.

using a metered dose inhaler (MDI). The various devices used to nebulize β-agonists all create a range of particle sizes that reach both the large airways (5–10-μm particles) and the small airways (1–5-μm particles). Particles larger than 10 μm impact on the oropharynx and approximately 10% are absorbed systemically.[42] The other major factor that determines aerosol delivery is the inspiratory flow rate. High flow rates increase impaction, leading to central deposition, and decrease deposition to peripheral airways.

MDIs are the most common delivery system for β-agonists and other anti-asthmatic aerosols. After the cannister is shaken and inverted, the stem is compressed and the activator releases particles of drug and propellant that are usually 30–50 μm in size. After evaporation, most particles decrease in size to 2.8–5.5 μm depending on the MDI used. Even with appropriate technique and slow inspiratory flow rates (30 L/min or a 5–10-second inspiration), only 10% of the dose is deposited in the lung. Studies show that even with instruction, MDIs cannot be effectively used in 30% of patients.[43] This group of patients should benefit from the use of a spacer. Spacers act as a holding chamber and enhance the effect of bronchodilators in patients with poor hand coordination. The decrease in the amount of oropharyngeal deposition of drug is helpful in preventing complications of inhaled corticosteroids but does not increase the amount of drug delivered when compared to a patient who properly uses a MDI.

In the interest of reducing the use of fluorocarbons as propellants dry powder inhalers (DPIs) have become more common. Some systems such as the albuterol rotahaler and cromolyn spinhaler have the disadvantage of requiring that the capsules be carried separately. DPIs have the advantage of being activated when the patient starts to inhale; however, they require flow rates of 80–120 L/min for maximal delivery of the drug to the airway. Children less than 5 years old cannot generate effective flow rates to use the DPI. Multidose DPIs have been developed and are undergoing clinical evaluation.[4]

β-agonists can also be delivered by nebulization with either a jet nebulizer or an ultrasonic nebulizer. These systems are frequently used in the Emergency Department. Radiolabelled studies show that only 10% of the medication is delivered to the airway with nebulization. This is the same percentage that is delivered with an MDI; however, much larger doses of drug are used with nebulization. A standard dose of albuterol 2.5 mg nebulized with a jet nebulizer will deliver 0.25 mg of drug. Two puffs with an MDI (0.1 mg/puff) will deliver 0.02 mg to the airways. Studies have shown that an MDI with a spacer is as effective as a jet nebulizer in treating asthma in the Emergency Department if equivalent doses are used.

β-Agonists can also be given orally or by injection. There are few data available to show the benefit of using these routes when patients with acute asthma are receiving adequate doses via nebulization. Subcutaneous injection may seem reasonable if there is a strong reason to suspect that the drug is not reaching the lower airway (e.g., because of severe mucus plugging). The oral route of delivery of β-agonists does offer the advantage of an increase in duration in patients who require chronic maintenance therapy for asthma. Slow-release preparation may be beneficial for patients with nocturnal symptoms or for those patients in whom compliance is a problem.

Glucocorticosteroids

Glucocorticosteroids act through the production of lipocortin, which has many beneficial effects on asthma. The mechanisms of action and the clinical use of corticosteroids have recently been reviewed.[44] Corticosteroids decrease inflammation, edema, and mucus production. They inhibit the production of histamine, prostaglandins, and leukotrienes. Glucocorticosteroids increase the number of β-receptors and improve receptor sensitivity. In addition, they inhibit the migration and function of eosinophils and neutrophils. Improved responsiveness to β-agonists occurs within 2 hours but an improved clinical response to glucocorticosteroids usually requires 4–12 hours.

Systemic corticosteroid treatment is recommended for acute severe asthma or for the treatment of impending episodes of severe asthma. Moderately severe asthma may also require systemic steroids. There are no data to show that the use of systemic steroids in patients with moderate asthma will promote a state of steroid dependency. Mild asthma can be treated with inhaled steroids and for many patients with moderate or severe asthma their steroid dose can be slowly tapered down and converted to inhaled steroids. Data suggest that doses of inhaled steroids have an equal effect to 15 mg/day of prednisone in patients with asthma.

In severe asthma requiring hospitalization, intravenous methylprednisolone 2 mg/kg (approximately 125 mg) should be administered every 6 hours for 24–48 hours. Then the dose should be decreased to 0.5–1 mg/kg every 6 hours until resolution of severe bronchospasm. This drug therapy can be changed to oral prednisone 1–2 mg/kg/day, which is also the recommended dose for treatment of impending episodes of severe asthma failing to respond to

Systemic corticosteroid treatment is recommended for the treatment of acute severe asthma or impending episodes of severe asthma. Moderately severe asthma may also require systemic steroids. There are no data that indicate that the use of systemic steroids in patients with moderate asthma will promote steroid dependency.

bronchodilators.[45] The duration of treatment depends on the patient's clinical response. Very short courses of systemic steroids are frequently effective and if less than 7–10 days in duration will rarely result in adrenal suppression. In general, short-course (1–2 week), high-dose (prednisone 1–2 mg/kg/day) systemic steroids do not produce serious toxicities. Patients receiving eight such courses of corticosteroids over 1 year exhibited a decrease in trabecular bone density equal to that of patients on daily or alternate-day steroids.[45] Therefore, even though short courses of corticosteroids have been shown to reduce hospitalization for asthma exacerbation, the clinician should always balance the benefit with the possible toxicities of systemic corticosteroid therapy.

Inhaled corticosteroids are becoming a first-line therapy for chronic asthma since inflammation appears to play a major role in the pathogenesis of asthma. The available inhaled corticosteroids, beclomethasone diproprionate, triamcinolone, and flunisolide, appear to have equal potency. Unfortunately, there are few clinical data comparing efficacy and toxicities. Patients derive increasing benefits from increasing doses but systemic toxicities can occur by exceeding the maximum recommended doses. Doses of beclomethasone greater than 800 µg/day cause measurable adrenal suppression. Maximal recommended doses for adults are equivalent to 1,600 µg/day for beclomethasone and triamcinolone or 2,000 µg/day for flunisolide. Patients requiring doses exceeding these levels should be monitored for adverse effects. Local adverse effects include candidiasis and dysphonia, which are dose dependent. The use of a spacer decreases local adverse effects.

Inhaled corticosteroids are becoming a first-line therapy for chronic asthma since inflammation appears to play a major role in the pathogenesis of asthma.

Methylxanthines

Methylxanthines, primarily theophylline, have been used in the treatment of asthma for over 50 years. Although theophylline has been considered a first-line drug in the treatment of status asthmaticus in the past, recent studies question its use in this setting.[46] This drug still has a major role in the treatment of chronic asthma and should be used as a second- or third-line drug in severe, acute asthma.

The mechanism of action of theophylline is not known. Theophylline is known to stimulate endogenous catecholamines and is a competitive antagonist to the bronchoconstrictor adenosine. Theophylline may produce bronchodilation by inhibiting the release of intracellular calcium.[4] Regardless of its mechanism of action, theophylline acts as a functional agonist and leads to bronchodilation unrelated to the cause of bronchoconstriction. Theophylline has sig-

Although theophylline has been considered a first-line drug in the treatment of status asthmaticus in the past, recent studies question its use in this setting.

nificant effects besides airway smooth muscle relaxation. Theophylline strengthens the contraction of a fatigued diaphragm, enhances mucociliary function, and decreases vascular permeability. Theophylline decreases the bronchospasm associated with the early and the late asthmatic response. There are no data, however, to show that theophylline reduces inflammation or prevents bronchial hyperreactivity.

One of the classic pharmacodynamic studies on theophylline was by Mintenko and Olgivie.[47] They demonstrated that theophylline produces a linear increase in pulmonary function with logarithmic increments in serum drug concentration. In their study, each log increment (i.e., from 0 to 5 μg/ml, 5 to 10 μg/ml, and 10 to 20 μg/ml) resulted in a 15–20% improvement in pulmonary function. The only flaw in their study was the attempt to extrapolate their data from chronic stable asthmatics to acutely ill asthmatics.[48] We know and understand that the dose–response curve for theophylline or other bronchodilators is not a static curve. When patients experience severe bronchospasm, the dose–response curve is shifted to the right. Although clinicians can easily increase the dose of β-agonists by a factor of 5–10 times the usual dose, the toxic–therapeutic range for theophylline is so narrow that significant increases lead to significant toxic side effects.

The majority of chronic stable asthmatics show significant bronchodilation with serum concentrations between 5 and 15 μg/ml. Most patients show minimal toxicity below a level of 15 μg/ml. Gastrointestinal (nausea and vomiting), cardiac (tachycardia and arrythmias), and central nervous system toxicity (reduced cerebral blood flow and seizures) occur with increasing serum concentrations. Adverse effects occur in approximately 18% at concentrations of 15–20 μg/ml, 60% at concentrations of 20–30 μg/ml, and as many as 80% at concentrations greater than 30 μg/ml.[34]

The serum half-life of theophylline in adults ranges from 6 to 12 hours, with significant interpatient variability. This large variability in clearance dictates routine monitoring of serum theophylline levels to prevent toxic side effects. Most outpatients should be treated with sustained-release preparations. These preparations can usually be dosed on a 12–24-hour schedule. Patients with rapid clearance rates may develop asthmatic symptoms prior to their next dose and require every 8 hours dosing.

Theophylline is cleared by the hepatic P-450 enzyme system. Dose reductions of 25–50% may be required with liver disease, congestive heart failure, febrile viral illness, and certain drugs. Common drugs that may decrease clearance include cimetidine, erythromycin, ciprofloxacin, proprano-lol, and oral contraceptives.

Theophylline should be considered for the treatment of chronic asthma that fails to respond to β-agonists and in-haled corticosteroids. It may be particularly useful in pa-tients with nocturnal asthma. The role of theophylline in hospitalized patients has not been clearly delineated. One recent review concluded that theophylline should be ad-ministered to hospitalized patients who fail optimal Emer-gency Department care.[48] Since this review, a double-blind, placebo-controlled trial of aminophylline for hospitalized asthmatics failed to demonstrate any benefit when amino-phylline was added to inhaled β-agonists and corticoste-roids. Until this issue is resolved, one approach would be to use theophylline in selected patients and monitor the theophylline level to ensure it remains at a nontoxic level between 10 and 15 μg/ml. The protocol at our institution is given in Table 3.

TABLE 3   Aminophylline Protocol

Loading Protocol: Obtain history of theophylline ingestion

None	Give 5-mg/kg loading dose over 30 min by constant IV infusion
Any amount	Obtain STAT serum concentration measurement *or* If asthma symptoms are severe and there is no clinical evidence of toxicity, give 2.5-mg/kg loading dose over 30 min by constant IV infusion

Infusion Protocol

	Aminophylline (mg/kg/hr)*
Healthy adults who smoke	0.6
Otherwise healthy nonsmoking adults	0.4–0.5
Cardiac decompensation and liver dysfunction	0.2

Monitoring Protocol: Obtain serum concentration 30 min after loading dose to ascertain if an additional loading dose is required

Concentration >25 μg/ml	Initial Concentration 10–20 μg/ml	Initial Concentration <10 μg/ml
Discontinue infusion until serum conc <20 μg/ml	Continue initial infusion	Give 1 mg/kg for each 2 μg/ml desired increase in serum conc

* Reduce dose by 25% for co-administration of cimetadine, erythromycin, ciprofloxacin, or oral contracep-tives.
† Target blood level for 10–15 μg/ml.

Anticholinergics

Anticholinergics were the first effective bronchodilators used for asthma. In the early 19th century, smoke from a plant of the *datura* species was used in Western medicine to treat asthma. Atropine sulfate, a tertiary ammonium compound, is completely absorbed from the lungs and the gastrointestinal tract. Concern over systemic side effects, particularly of the central nervous system, limited the widespread use of atropine in the treatment of obstructive airways disease. The recent development of quaternary ammonium derivatives such as ipratropium bromide (Atrovent) has renewed interest in these compounds. Ipratropium bromide has the advantages over earlier anticholinergics of being poorly absorbed across mucosal surfaces, poorly penetrating the blood–brain barrier, and not producing the decrease in mucociliary clearance seen with atropine.

Anticholinergic agents inhibit muscarinic receptors and decrease vagal parasympathetic bronchial tone. Unlike β-agonists or theophylline, which reduce bronchoconstriction regardless of the cause, ipratropium and atropine produce bronchodilation only in cholinergic-mediated bronchoconstriction. There are a number of triggers (i.e., exercise, sulfur dioxide, allergens, emotional stress) and mediators (i.e., histamine, prostaglandins) that produce bronchoconstriction via vagal stimulation.[34] Therefore, anticholinergic drugs are more dependent on the mechanism of bronchospasm than other agents. Anticholinergics appear to be as effective as β-agonists in reversing the bronchospasm of chronic bronchitis; however, a critical review of the 18 clinical trails of anticholinergics in acute severe asthma concluded that these agents should be considered second-line therapy for acute asthma.[49]

Most studies demonstrated anticholinergics produce an additional 20–25% improvement in FEV_1 over β-agonists alone. This improvement was not associated with an improvement in clinical outcome. In those studies in which patients received only anticholinergics or β-agonists, bronchospasm was more consistently and completely reversed by β-agonists. Only one of eight studies comparing anticholinergics to β-agonists as initial therapy in acute asthma reported equivalent results.[50] All the other studies showed that anticholinergics were less effective bronchodilators in the initial therapy of asthma.[49] Five studies in adults compared β-agonist alone with the combination of β-agonist and anticholinergics.[51–55] One study found no difference between the two treatments but did suggest a longer duration of action for the combination.[51] The other four studies

Most studies have demonstrated that anticholinergics produce an additional 20–25% improvement in FEV_1 over beta agonists alone. This improvement is not associated with an improvement in clinical outcome.

all reported significantly greater bronchodilation with the combination of anticholinergics and β-agonist. This difference was most striking in the group of patients with severe obstruction (peak expiratory flow rate [PEFR] less than 35% predicted) and the combination of anticholinergics and β-agonist should be considered in this subset of patients.

The anticholinergics have a longer duration of action than the β-agonists that are currently available. The onset of action and the time to peak bronchodilation is considerably slower than with β-agonists. Therefore, anticholinergics should never be administered for acute asthma without β-agonists. Additionally, the studies of anticholinergics in acute asthma used significantly higher doses (equivalent to 10–20 puffs of ipratropium) than those recommended for chronic therapy. The development of anticholinergics that selectively block the smooth muscle (M_3) receptor may increase their usefulness in the therapy of asthma.

Cromolyn Sodium

Cromolyn sodium was first released in the United States for treatment of asthma in the early 1970s. This drug was initially recommended only for steroid-dependent asthmatics despite the fact that it is undoubtedly the least toxic drug available in the treatment of asthma. Cromolyn is now considered an effective drug in managing patients with mild-to-moderate chronic asthma.[4]

Despite intensive research, the mechanism of action of cromolyn is not completely known. Its primary mode of action is believed to be stabilization of mast cells.[56] Cromolyn also inhibits activation of neutrophils, monocytes, and PAF. Some studies have demonstrated an acute improvement in pulmonary function tests with inhalation of cromolyn;[57–59] however, this finding is not consistently seen.[60–61] In addition, cromolyn potentiates β-agonist-induced smooth muscle relaxation in animal studies.[4] Cromolyn has been shown to inhibit the early and late asthmatic response with antigen challenge[62] as well as exercise induced asthma.[63] Long-term prophylaxis with cromolyn prevents bronchial hyperreactivity to allergens and, to a lesser degree, to histamine challenge.[4] These studies suggest cromolyn inhibits the inflammatory response of asthma.

Cromolyn is indicated for the prevention of symptoms in mild-to-moderate asthma regardless of etiology. Although it appears to be more effective in children and in "allergic" asthmatics, overall approximately 50–60% of asthma will be adequately controlled with cromolyn.[62] Cromolyn is effective in the prevention of EIA and should be used in this setting when β-agonists fail to prevent symp-

Cromolyn is indicated for the prevention of symptoms in chronic mild to moderate asthma regardless of etiology. Although it appears to be more effective in children and in "allergic" asthmatics, overall approximately 50–60% of asthma is adequately controlled with cromolyn.

toms or when exercise induces a late asthmatic response. Cromolyn may allow for the reduction of corticosteroids, but it is primarily indicated for prophylaxis of less severe disease.

Cromolyn may be administered as a 20-mg powdered capsule via spinhaler, as a 1% solution containing cromolyn 20 mg in 2 ml of distilled water via a nebulizer, or as a pressurized MDI that delivers cromolyn 1 mg. The starting dose is 20 mg by spinhaler or nebulizer or 2 inhalations by MDI four times daily. When symptoms are controlled, the frequency can be reduced to three times a day, then twice daily. If the results of a trial of cromolyn are equivocal at 4 weeks, the trial should be extended to 8 to 12 weeks. Although the older powder formulation of cromolyn should not be administered during an acute exacerbations of asthma, this is not necessary with the solution or the MDI.

Other Antiinflammatory Drugs

Methotrexate. Methotrexate has been used in the management of chronic rheumatoid arthritis for many years. Recent studies by Mullarkey et al. show a beneficial effect of low-dose (15 mg weekly) methotrexate in steroid-dependent asthmatics.[64] A recent double-blind, placebo-controlled study was not able to replicate these findings.[65] Whether the differences in these results relate to differences in the study population must be determined. Long-term side effects of methotrexate include cirrhosis and pulmonary fibrosis. At this time, methotrexate should be reserved for patients with very severe asthma.

Gold. Gold injections (chysotherapy) has also been used for the treatment of rheumatoid arthritis. In Japan, similar therapy used in steroid-dependent asthmatics has been shown to reduce the amount of prednisone needed to control the disease.[66] Recent uncontrolled studies support the concept that orally administered gold (6 mg/day) has a steroid-sparing effect.[67] Controlled studies will have to be performed to establish the role of gold in the treatment of asthma.

SUMMARY

Asthma is a chronic inflammatory disease characterized by excessive reactivity of the bronchial tree. This excessive reactivity appears to be linked to the extent of inflammation in the airways. The goal in the management of acute asthma is to restore pulmonary function and reverse the patient's symptoms. Once the patient is evaluated in the Emergency Department or hospitalized, an additional goal is to prevent respiratory failure or death caused by inadequate assessment or inadequate therapy. In chronic asthma, therapy should be directed at the prevention of symptoms through the use of bronchodilators and anti-inflammatory drugs. Patient education and self-monitoring are fundamental in the optimal care of asthmatic patients.

References

1. Fleming DM, Cromble DL: Prevalence of asthma and hay fever in England and Wales. Br Med J 294:279, 1987

2. Jackson R, Sears MR, Beaglehole R et al: International trends in asthma mortality. Chest 94(5):914, 1988

3. Sly RM: Increase in death from asthma. Ann Allergy 53:20, 1984

4. Kaliner MA, Barnes PJ, Persson CGA (eds): Asthma: its pathology and treatment. Marcel Dekker, New York, 1991

5. American Thoracic Society Committee on Diagnostic Standards: Definitions and classification of chronic bronchitis, asthma and pulmonary emphysema. Am Rev Respir Dis 85:762, 1962

6. Scientific Assembly on Allergy and Clinical Immunology subcommittee: definition of asthma. ATS News 5, 1982

7. Parker SR, Mellins RB, Sogn DD: NHLBI workshop summary. Asthma education: a national strategy. Am Rev Respir Dis 140:848, 1989

8. Broder I, Higgins MW, Matthews KP et al: Epidemiology of asthma and allergic rhinitis in a total community. Tecumseh, Michigan, III. Second survey of the community. J Allergy Clin Immunol 53:127, 1974

9. Dodge RR, Burrows B: The prevalence and incidence of asthma and asthma-like symptoms in a general population sample. Am Rev Respir Dis 122:567, 1980

10. Schachter EN, Doyle GA, Beck GJ: A prospective study of asthma in a rural population. Chest 85:623, 1984

11. Weiss ST, Speizer FE: The epidemiology of asthma: risk factors and natural history. p. 14. In Weiss EB, Segal MS, Stein M (eds): Bronchial asthma: mechanisms and therapeutics. 2nd Ed. Little, Brown, Boston, 1985

12. Benatar SA: Fatal asthma. N Engl J Med 314:423, 1986

13. Juniper EF, Frith PA, Hargreave FE: Airway responsiveness to histamine and methacholine: relationship to minimum treatment to control symptoms of asthma. Thorax 36:575, 1981

14. Woodcock AJ, Salome CM, Yan K: The shape of the dose-response curve to histamine in asthmatic and normal subjects. Am Rev Respir Dis 130:71, 1984

15. Barnes PJ: New concepts in the pathogenesis of bronchial hyperresponsiveness and asthma. J Allergy Clin Immunol 83:1013, 1989

16. Laitinen LA, Heino M, Laitinen A et al: Damage of the airway epithelium and bronchial reactivity in patients with asthma. Am Rev Respir Dis 131:599, 1985

17. Beasley R, Roche WR, Roberts JA, Holgate ST: Cellular events in the bronchi in mild asthma and after bonchial provocation. Am Rev Respir Dis 139:806, 1989

18. Jeffrey PK, Wardlaw AJ, Nelson FC et al: Bronchial biopsies in asthma. An ultrastructural, quantitative study and correlation with hyperreactivity. Am Rev Respir Dis 140:1745, 1989

19. Kaliner M: Asthma and mast cell activation. J Allergy Clin Immunol 83:510, 1989

20. Church MK, Hiroi J: Inhibition of IgE-dependent histamine release from human dispersed lung mast cells by antiallergic drugs and salbutamol. Br J Pharmacol 90:421, 1987

21. De Monchy JGR, Kauffman HF, Venge P et al: Bronchoalveolar eosinophils during allergen-induced late asthmatic reactions. Am Rev Respir Dis 131:373, 1985

22. Wardlaw AJ, Chung KF, Moqbel R et al: Cellular changes in blood and bronchoalveolar lavage (BAL) and bronchial responsiveness after inhaled PAF in man. Am Rev Respir Dis 137(Suppl):283, 1988

23. Gleich GJ: The eosinophil and bronchial asthma: current understanding. J Allergy Clin Immunol 85:422, 1990

24. Wardlaw AJ, Moqbel R, Cromwell O, Kay AB: Platelet-activating factor: a potent chemotactic and chemokinetic factor for human eosinophils. J Clin Invest 78:1701, 1986

25. Joseph M, Tonnel AB, Tarpier G, Capron A: Involvement of immunoglobulin E in the secretory process of alveolar macrophages from asthmatic patients. J Clin Invest 71:221, 1983

26. Godard P, Chainteuil J, Damon M et al: Functional assessment of alveolar macrophages: comparison of cells from asthmatics and normal subjects. J Allergy Clin Immunol 70:80, 1982

27. Frew AJ, Moqbel R, Azzawi M et al: T-lymphocytes and eosinophils in allergen-induced late-phase asthmatic response in the guinea pig. Am Rev Resp Dis 141:407, 1990

28. Barnes PJ, Chung KF, Page CP: Inflammatory mediators in asthma. Pharmacol Rev 40:49, 1988

29. Barnes PJ, Chung KF, Page CP: Platelet-activating factor as a medicator of allergic disease [Review]. J Allergy Clin Immunol 81:919, 1988

30. Chung KF, Barnes PJ: PAF antagonists: their therapeutic potential in asthma. Drugs 35:93, 1988

31. Barnes PJ: Neural control of human airways in health and disease. Am Rev Respir Dis 134:1289, 1986

32. Minette PA, Barnes PJ: Prejunctional inhibitory muscarinic receptors on cholinergic nerves in human and guinea pig airways. J Appl Physiol 64:2532, 1988

33. Barnes PJ: Neuropeptides in human airways: function and clinical implications. Am Rev Respir Dis 136:S77, 1987

34. Jenne JS, Murphy SA (eds): Drug therapy for asthma: research and clinical practice. Marcel Dekker, New York, 1987

35. Weiss EB, Segal MS, Stein M (eds): Bronchial asthma: mechanisms and therapeutics. 2nd Ed. Little, Brown, Boston, 1985

36. Anderson SD: Exercise-induced asthma: the state of the art. Chest 87(suppl):191, 1985

37. Lee TH, Nagakura T, Paplageorgioun N et al: Exercise-induced late asthmatic reactions wiith neutrophil chemotactic activity. N Engl J Med 308:1502, 1983

38. Ballard RD, Martin RJ: Nocturnal asthma. Semin Resp Med 8:302, 1987

39. Platts-Mills TAE, Mitchell EB, Nock P et al: Reduction of bronchial hyperreactivity during prolonged allergen avoidance. Lancet 2:675, 1982

40. Ohman JL: Allergen immunotherapy in asthma: evidence for efficacy. J Allergy Clin Immunol 84:133, 1989

41. Kelly HW: New 82-agonist aerosols. Clin Pharm 4:393, 1985

42. Kim CS, Eldridge MA, Sackner MA: Oropharyngeal deposition and delivery aspects of metered-dose inhaler aerosols. Am Rev Respir Dis 135:157, 1987

43. Newman SP: Aerosol deposition considerations in inhalation therapy. Chest 88(Suppl):152, 1985

44. Sertl K, Clark T, Kaliner M (eds): Corticosteroids: their biologic mechanisms and application to the treatment of asthma. Am Rev Respir Dis 141(Suppl):S1, 1990

45. Kelly HW, Murphy S: Corticosteroids for acute severe asthma. Drug Intell Clin Pharm 25:72, 1991

46. Self TH, Abou-Shala N, Burns R et al: Inhaled albuterol and oral prednisone therapy in hospitalized adult asthmatics: does animophylline add any benefit? Chest 98:1317, 1990

47. Mintenko PA, Olgivie RI: Rational intravenous doses of theophylline. N Engl J Med 289:600, 1973

48. Kelly HW, Murphy S: Should we stop using theophylline for the treatment of the hospitalized patient with status asthmaticus? Drug Intel Clin Pharm 23:995, 1989

49. Kelly HW, Murphy S: Should anticholinergics be used in acute severe asthma? Drug Intell Clin Pharm 24:409, 1990

50. Ward MJ, Fentem PH, Smith WHR, Davies D: Ipratropium bromide in acute asthma. Br Med J 282:598, 1981

51. Higgins RM, Stradling JR, Lane DJ: Should ipratropium bromide be added to beta-agonists in treatment of acute severe asthma. Chest 94:718, 1988

52. Watson WA, Becker AB, Simons FER: Ipratropium solution (Ipr) versus fenoterol solution (Fen) versus the combined solutions (Comb) in the treatment of acute asthma in children (abstract). J Allergy Clin Immunol 79:151, 1987

53. Rebuck AS, Chapman KR, Abboud R et al: Nebulized anti-cholinergic and sympathomimetic treatment of asthma and chronic obstructive airways disease in the emergency room. Am J Med 82:59, 1987

54. Lew DB, Herrod HG, Crawford LV: The effect of adding atropine sulfate (As) to a maximal dose of Bronkosol (B) inhalation in pediatric status asthma (Sa) (Abstract). J Allergy Clin Immunol 81:316, 1988

55. O'Driscoll BR, Horsley MG, Taylor RJ et al: Nebulized salbutamol with and without ipratropium bromide in acute airflow obstruction. Lancet 1:1418, 1989

56. Orr TSC, Cox JSG: Disodium cromoglycate: an inhibitor of mast cell degranulation and histamine release induced by phospholipase A. Nature 223:197, 1969

57. Hughes D, Mindorff C, Levinson H: The immediate effect of sodium cromoglycate on the airways. Ann Allergy 48:6, 1982

58. Weiner P, Greif J, Fireman E: Bronchodilating effect of cromolyn sodium in asthmatic patients at rest and following exercise. Ann Allergy 53:186, 1984

59. Horn CR, Jones RM, Lee D, Brennan SR: Bronchodilator effect of disodium cromoglycate administered as a dry powder in exercise-induced asthma. Br J Pharmacol 18:798, 1984

60. Chung JTN, Jones RS: Bronchodilator effects of sodium cromoglycate and its clinical implications. Br Med J 11:1033, 1979

61. Hasham F, Kennedy JD, Jones RS: Actions of salbutamol, disodium cromolgycate and placebo administered as aerosols in acute asthma. Arch Dis Child 56:722, 1981

62. Murphy S, Kelly HW: Cromolyn sodium: a review of mechanisms and clinical use in asthma. Drug Intell Clin Pharm 21:22, 1987

63. Davies SE: Effect of disodium cromoglycate on exercise-induced asthma. Br Med J 3:593, 1968

64. Mullarkey MF, Blumenstein BA, Andrade WP et al: Methotrexate in the treatment of corticoste-roid-dependent asthma: a double-blind crossover study. N Engl J Med 318:603, 1988

65. Erzurum SC, Leff JA et al: Lack of benefit of Methotrexate in severe, steroid-dependent asthma. A double-blind, placebo-controlled study. Ann Intern Med 114:353, 1991

66. Muranaka M, Mivamoto T, Shida T et al: Gold salt in the treatment of bronchial asthma—a double-blind study. Ann Allergy 40:132, 1978

67. Bernstein DI, Bernstein IL, Bodenheimer SS, Pietrusko RG: An open study of auranofin in the treatment of steroid-dependent asthma. J Allergy Clin Immunol 81:6, 1988

TRANSPLANTATION FOR OBSTRUCTIVE LUNG DISEASE

STEPHANIE M. LEVINE, MD
CHARLES L. BRYAN, MD

With the advent of improved immunosuppressive therapy, the past decade has seen a flourish in solid organ transplantation. In the early 1980s, human heart–lung transplantation (HLT) was successfully performed for the treatment of pulmonary vascular disease.[1] Following this procedure, single-lung transplantation (SLT) for the treatment of end-stage interstitial lung disease was developed.[2] More recently, the technique of double-lung transplantation (DLT) has come into existence. The first part of this chapter will present a review of the specific indications and surgical techniques for SLT, HLT, and DLT followed by sections on recipient selection and evaluation, donor evaluation, recipient–donor compatibility criteria, and postoperative surveillance tests. This chapter will concentrate specifically on results of transplantation for end-stage obstructive lung disease due to panlobular emphysema, centrilobular emphysema, and cystic fibrosis (CF). Finally, we will conclude with a discussion of some of the remaining problems facing lung transplantation today.

SINGLE LUNG TRANSPLANTATION

History

Human SLT dates back to 1963 when Dr. James Hardy at the University of Mississippi performed the first SLT on a 58-year-old man with bronchogenic carcinoma.[3] The patient survived for 18 days. In the next two decades, approximately 40 SLTs were attempted without success.[4] The major reasons for the poor outcome in these patients included graft rejection and anastomotic complications. With the advent of cyclosporin A and other immunosuppressive agents, the problem of rejection has substantially decreased. In addition, newer surgical techniques, including the bronchial telescoping technique, have resulted in a dramatic decrease in anastomotic problems. In 1983, the To-

The major reasons for poor outcome in transplantation patients have included graft rejection and anastomotic complications; cyclosporin A and other immunosuppressive agents have substantially decreased the problem of rejection.

ronto Lung Transplant Group conducted the first long-term, successful SLT in a patient with idiopathic pulmonary fibrosis.[2] Since then more than 350 SLTs have been performed worldwide. In 1990, the International Registry for Lung Transplantation reported a 1- and 2-year survival rate of 78% and 74%, respectively, following SLT. These figures are a remarkable improvement over the early 1970s, when only 1 out of 40 lung transplant recipients had survived long enough to achieve hospital discharge. If conditions affecting transplantation continue to improve at the same rate, survival could reach 90% by the year 2000.[5]

Indications

SLT has been performed in patients with end-stage restrictive lung disease secondary to fibrotic lung disease. The indications have recently been expanded to include patients with nonseptic end-stage obstructive lung disease.

The current indications for SLT are shown in Table 1. Until 1989, SLT had been performed in patients with end-stage restrictive lung disease secondary to idiopathic pulmonary fibrosis (IPF) or the other listed causes of fibrotic lung disease. More recently, indications for SLT have been expanded to include patients with nonseptic end-stage obstructive lung disease.[6,7] It is important to emphasize that patients with CF, bronchiectasis, or other forms of septic obstructive lung disease cannot be considered for SLT. This is because the remaining native septic lung, particularly when subjected to immunosuppression, could infect the new transplanted lung.

Previously, SLT for the treatment of obstructive lung disease was not considered possible. There was concern that the placement of a transplanted lung with normal vascular resistance and compliance in parallel circuit with an emphysematous lung with high compliance and high vascular resistance would result in ventilation/perfusion (V/Q) inequality.[8,9] The conventional theory held that the majority of the perfusion would be distributed to the transplant while the emphysematous native lung would receive the majority of the ventilation, resulting in potential hyperinflation and compression of the newly transplanted lung graft.[8] In fact, this was the result in two patients with emphysema undergoing SLT in the late 1970s.[9] Both patients succumbed to rejection and/or infection of the transplanted lung. However, both animal studies and a human case report (also from the 1970s) determined that SLT for the treatment of emphysema was possible as long as the transplanted lung graft was free of rejection, infection, or other causes of alveolar infiltrates.[10] In 1988, the first successful SLT for the treatment of pulmonary emphysema was performed in France.[11] In January 1989, Dr. J. Kent Trinkle at the University of Texas Health Science Center at San Antonio (UTHSC-SA) performed the first successful SLT for em-

TABLE 1   Indications for SLT

Restrictive
  Idiopathic pulmonary
    fibrosis
  Sarcoidosis
  Scleroderma (limited)
  Asbestosis
  Silicosis
Obstructive
  Emphysema
  α_1-ATD
  Lymphangioleiomyo-
    matosis
  Bronchiolitis obliterans
  Eosinophilic granuloma
Primary pulmonary
  hypertension

physema in North America on a 45-year-old man with α_1-antitrypsin deficiency (α_1-ATD).[12] Washington University in St. Louis soon followed in March 1989[13] by performing a SLT on a 60-year-old man with chronic obstructive pulmonary disease (COPD).

The most recent proposed indication for SLT is primary pulmonary hypertension (PPH). Previously, SLT was thought to be contraindicated for PPH because of the potential V/Q mismatch produced by placing a native lung with a fixed high vascular resistance and normal pulmonary compliance in parallel with a transplanted lung with normal compliance and normal vascular resistance.[1] In this situation, ventilation would theoretically be split equally between the two lungs while the majority of perfusion would go to the transplanted lung. At UTHSC-SA, we have performed three SLTs for PPH.[14] Despite the above predicted V/Q pattern, which we did in fact find in our three patients, our patients were able to maintain normal arterial oxygenation and were able to perform activities of daily living without compromise. However, during episodes of biopsy-proven rejection, there was a further shift of ventilation to the native lung without a corresponding change in perfusion. This severe V/Q mismatch resulted in marked hypoxemia and resting arterial desaturation. These findings suggest that DLT is a better procedure for patients with PPH than SLT.

The Choice of Side

The choice of side to transplant in SLT is based on a number of factors. If the recipients pleural space has been previously breached by open-lung biopsy or pneumothorax with chemical or surgical pleurodesis, the contralateral hemithorax should be chosen. If preoperative V/Q scanning shows that one lung functions significantly better than the other lung, the less functional lung should be transplanted. If the recipient has had no previous surgery and the lungs function equally, the left side has traditionally been chosen for transplantation. This is because the surgery is technically easier to perform on the left side.[12] It is easier to clamp the left atrium proximal to the pulmonary vein on the left and it is possible to leave a larger donor atrial cuff and longer recipient bronchus. For these reasons, at our institution, if the patient is undergoing SLT for end-stage interstitial lung disease, the left side is preferred.

Some transplant surgeons prefer the right side for transplantation in obstructive disease.[12] They believe that left SLTs used in obstructive patients allow the right hyperexpanded lung to compress the left lung since the right lung

The most recent proposed indication for SLT is primary pulmonary hypertension.

Pulmonary function testing, exercise oximetry, and V/Q lung scanning results do not support a functional difference between the right and left graft position for the treatment of obstructive lung disease.

is limited inferiorly by the liver. However, if a right graft is used the native left lung can expand inferiorly without compressing the right lung graft.[12] This concept is seemingly apparent on chest radiograph (Fig. 1). On the left is a posteroanterior chest radiograph of an emphysematous patient with a left lung graft on the right is an emphysematous patient with a right lung graft. Note the apparent compression of the transplanted left lung by the native hyperinflated right lung. In contrast, this compression is less dramatic when the transplant is placed in the right position. These findings are more cosmetic than real. The results of pulmonary function testing, exercise oximetry, and V/Q lung scanning do not support a functional difference between the right and left graft position for the treatment of obstructive lung diseases.[15]

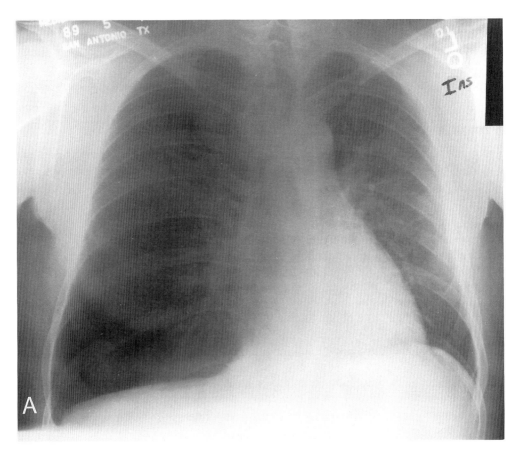

FIG. 1   (A) Posteroanterior radiograph of an α_1-ATD patient following a left-sided transplant. (*Figure continues*)

Surgical Technique[12]

The donor lung is usually harvested at the time of cardiac harvest via a median sternotomy incision. The pulmonary veins along with a 5-mm cuff of left atrium are detached from the heart. The pulmonary artery is transected from the main pulmonary artery and the mainstem bronchus is transected between two staple lines, as shown in Figure 2 (in this case a left lung harvest). Following preservation of the donor lung graft in Euro-Collins solution (a crystalloid solution with intracellular electrolyte composition) at 4°C, the lung is transported to the recipient site. The recipient surgery is performed through a posterolateral thoracotomy incision. The donor pulmonary vein is anastomosed end-to-end to the recipient's left atrium (Fig. 3). This is followed by suturing the bronchial anastomosis, the technical details

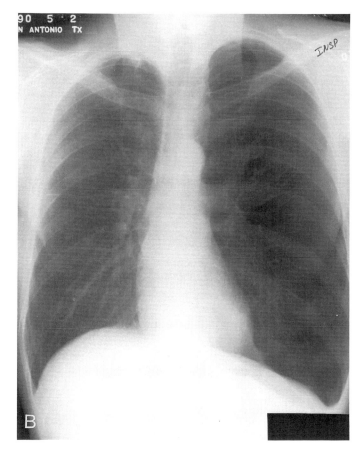

FIG. 1 (*continued*) (B) Radiograph of an α_1-ATD patient following right-sided transplant (above right).

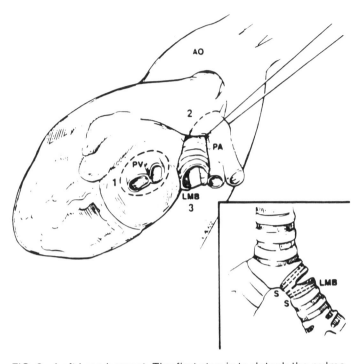

FIG. 2   Left lung harvest. The first step is to detach the pulmonary veins (PV) from the heart along with a 5 mm cuff of left atrium. The second step is to transect the pulmonary artery (PA) from the main PA. The third step is to transect the left main bronchus (LMB) between two staple lines, as shown in the inset. From Calhoon JH, Grover FL, Gibbons WJ et al: Single lung transplantation: alternative indications. J Thoracic Cardiovasc Surg 101:816–825, 1991. With permission.

of which vary among institutions. At some transplant centers, the anastomosis is sewn end-to-end and then a piece of omentum with an intact vascular pedicle is brought up and wrapped around the anastomosis in order to promote bronchial revascularization. It is important to remember that the lungs are the only organs that are transplanted without complete vascular reanastomosis (i.e., the bronchial circulation of the recipient and donor lungs are not anastomosed). This lack of revascularization of the bronchial circulation is the major factor in the numerous anastomotic complications plaguing lung transplantation, including bronchial dehiscence, bronchial stenosis, and bronchial infection. At other institutions, the bronchial anastomosis is performed by a telescoping technique (Fig. 4). The recipient and donor bronchi are overlapped by approximately one cartilaginous depth using insoluble 4-0 Prolene sutures. Thus, the intact bronchial circulation of the recipient is better able to supply the donor bronchus. Using this telescoping technique, our institution has had no bronchial

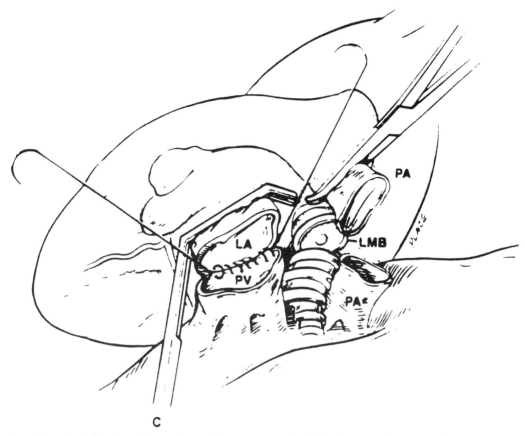

C

FIG. 3   Single left lung transplant with anastomosis of the donor pulmonary veins (PV) to the recipient left atrium (LA). PA, Pulmonary artery; LMB, left main bronchus. From Calhoon JH, Grover FL, Gibbons WJ et al: Single lung transplantation: alternative indications. J Thoracic Cardiovasc Surg 101:816–825, 1991. With permission.

anastomotic complications.[16] In contrast, the end-to-end anastomotic technique, even in conjunction with the omental wrap, has resulted in many reported cases of bronchial infection, stenosis requiring stent placement, and dehiscence. Finally, the surgery is completed by an end-to-end anastomosis of the donor and recipient pulmonary arteries (Fig. 5). The lung graft is allowed to perfuse in retrograde fashion via the pulmonary vein to allow egress of intra-arteriolar air.

HEART-LUNG TRANSPLANTATION

History

Attempts at human HLT date back to the 1960s, when in 1968 Cooley attempted an HLT in an infant with atrioventricular venous canal defect and pulmonary hypertension. She survived only 14 hours.[17] In 1969, Lillehei performed

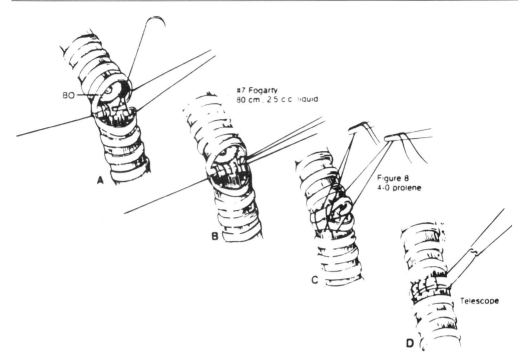

FIG. 4 Bronchial anastomosis. (A) 4-0 Prolene traction sutures are placed at each end of the membranous portion of the bronchus. The first traction suture is tied and a continuous posterior suture line is placed before the second traction suture is tied. (B) The posterior suture line has been completed and the bronchial blocker, a no 7 Fogarty catheter 80 cm long with a 2.5-ml liquid balloon, is shown in place. (C) The anterior bronchial anastomosis is completed by placing figure-of-eight 4-0 Prolene sutures around the cartilages. (D) After the anterior sutures are tied, the bronchus naturally telescopes to a depth of one cartilage. From Calhoon JH, Grover FL, Gibbons WJ et al: Single lung transplantation: alternative indications. J Thoracic Cardiovasc Surg 101:816–825, 1991. With permission.

a HLT on a 43-year-old man with emphysema. He survived 8 days following the transplantation.[18] In 1971, a third HLT was performed and this patient survived 23 days before succumbing to an anastomotic fistula and nosocomial pneumonia.[19] In 1981, after cyclosporin A had been shown to prevent renal allograft rejection, an experimental clinical trial of HLT began at Stanford University.[20] The first patient was a woman with PPH who survived for 5 years.[1] Since that time, 761 patients have undergone HLT worldwide.[21] At Stanford University, where the majority of HLTs in the United States have been performed, the recent 1- and 2-year survival rates are both 86%.[21] In the United Kingdom, these figures are 78% and 68%, respectively.

Indications

The current indications for HLT are shown in Table 2. As stated previously, the initial indications for HLT were PPH or hypertension secondary to congenital heart disease.

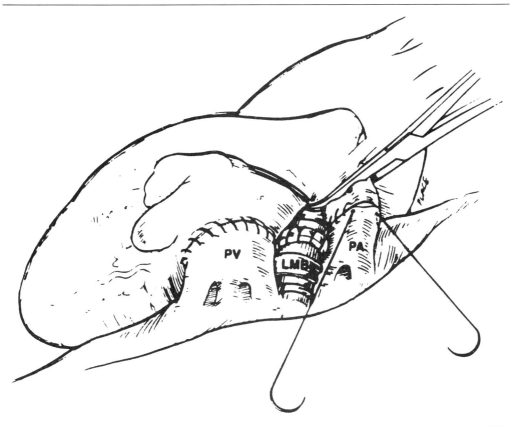

FIG. 5 Completion of a single left lung transplant with a running 4-0 Prolene suture of the pulmonary artery (PA). PV, Pulmonary vein; LMB, left main bronchus. From Calhoon JH, Grover FL, Gibbons WJ et al: Single lung transplantation: alternative indications. J Thoracic Cardiovasc Surg 101:816–825, 1991. With permission.

More recently, indications for HLT have been expanded to include patients with intrinsic pulmonary disease with secondary pulmonary hypertension. Patients with primary lung disease and unrelated but significant cardiovascular disease are also possible candidates for HLT.

There are several disadvantages with HLT as opposed to SLT for end-stage lung disease. One problem is the limited availability of donor organs. It would be preferable to use SLT as opposed to HLT when treating primary lung disease without associated cardiac disease. This would allow for the heart and remaining lung to be used in other patients

TABLE 2   Indications for HLT

Primary pulmonary hypertension with significant right ventricular dysfunction
Pulmonary disease with noncorrectable Eisenmenger's syndrome
Pulmonary disease with unrelated cardiac disease

on the transplant waiting list. Prior to the common use of SLT, organ maximization was attempted by the use of the domino procedure.[22] In this procedure, the en block HLT was transplanted into the recipient patient and the recipient's native heart was transplanted into a second patient requiring only a heart graft. Opponents believe that the domino procedure unnecessarily subjects the patient with lung disease to a larger surgical procedure, increases the amount of foreign material in the chest, and "gives away" his good heart.

A major problem with HLT is the significant incidence of chronic graft rejection or obliterative bronchiolitis.

A second major problem with HLT is the significant incidence of chronic graft rejection or obliterative bronchiolitis (OB). This is the major cause of morbidity following HLT and developed in about 50% of patients undergoing HLT in the early 1980s.[20] With augmented three-drug immunosuppression, the incidence of OB has decreased to approximately 20–30% in HLT recipients.[23,24] Initially it appeared that OB would be less common in SLT recipients. However, OB is now well described in SLT and perhaps as time progresses, may be nearly as common as is seen in HLT.[25–28]

Finally, if the first lung graft in a patient with intrinsic lung disease fails, a second SLT can be performed on the contralateral side. A second transplant can be performed in HLT recipients as well, but the second procedure is technically more difficult because of pleural adhesions and mediastinal cicatrization.

Surgical Technique

The donor organs are removed via a median sternotomy incision. The superior vena cava is ligated and transected, and the inferior vena cava and the aorta are cross-clamped. The heart is perfused with cardioplegic solution. Following this, the organs are flushed with prostacyclin and Euro-Collins solution. The recipient surgery is performed via a median sternotomy with the use of cardiopulmonary bypass. The organs are implanted by anastomosing the trachea approximately 2 cm above the carina, the right atria, and the donor and recipient ascending aorta.

DOUBLE LUNG TRANSPLANTATION

History and Indications

For certain indications, such as septic pulmonary disease due to CF and/ or bronchiectasis, only DLT is possible.

DLT began in 1984 when the Toronto Lung Transplant Group performed the first successful procedure in North America on a patient with end-stage obstructive lung disease.[29] Since that time, SLT has become the procedure of choice for end-stage nonseptic obstructive lung disease.

However, there are certain indications for which only DLT is possible, such as septic pulmonary disease due to CF and/or bronchiectasis. SLT in this patient group would allow a large residual focus of infection in the native lung to produce infection in the lung graft and/or sepsis. This problem would be further compounded by posttransplant immunosuppression. The current indications for DLT are listed in Table 3. Based on our results for SLT in PPH,[30] it now appears that DLT may be the procedure of choice for PPH because of problems with V/Q mismatch during rejection.

Surgical Technique

There are two ways of performing the DLT procedure, en bloc transplantation and sequential double SLT. Initially DLT was performed through a median sternotomy incision and the lungs were removed en bloc. The recipient surgery was performed using cardiopulmonary bypass by creating three anastomoses: one tracheal, one arterial, and one atrial. Problems with the en bloc DLT procedure included airway complications as reported with SLT. Three of six patients undergoing en bloc DLT for end-stage emphysema developed anastomotic complications.[29] These complications included a stricture in one patient, partial dehiscence in a second patient, and ischemic necrosis and dehiscence of the membranous wall of the donor trachea in a third patient. The latter patient required YAG laser therapy for tracheal stenosis followed by a tracheal stent placement.[29] In a larger series, there has been a 43% incidence of early and late airway complications due to en bloc DLT.[31]

Anastomotic complications in patients undergoing DLT should be more common than those occurring following SLT since the donor tracheobronchial circulation is interrupted. In contrast, with SLT, only a small segment of the donor mainstem bronchus is not vascularized.

More recently, sequential double SLTs have been performed.[32] In this procedure, the recipient surgery is performed through bilateral thoracotomies with transverse sternotomy. Two bronchial anastomoses and four vascular anastomoses are required. This procedure eliminates the need for bypass, and also reduces the incidence of postoperative airway complications since more recipient bronchi with their own bronchial vascularization are retained.

RECIPIENT SELECTION

Due to the limited availability of donor organs, recipient selection is a crucial part of the transplant process. It is important that the correct operative procedure be matched

TABLE 3   Indications for DLT

Cystic fibrosis
Bronchiectasis
? Primary pulmonary
    hypertension

Selection criteria vary between transplant centers, but some general medical and psychosocial requirements apply for all potential transplant recipients.

to the recipients need, in order to maximize the use of available donor organs as described above. If the patient meets the indications for a transplant procedure, the patient should be referred to a center performing that particular procedure. Most transplant programs now perform SLT and more recently, sequential bilateral SLT is available at many centers.

Selection criteria vary between transplant centers but some general medical and psychosocial requirements apply for all potential transplant recipients (Table 4). No single criterion is totally prohibitive. After meeting indication criteria for end-stage lung disease, the patient should have end-stage lung disease with an anticipated life expectancy of less than 18 months. It is important not to perform the surgery when the patient's symptoms are only mild to moderate; however, the transplant should not be delayed until the patient has deteriorated to a state where surgery would likely be unsuccessful.

Age criteria also differ between transplant centers, but at the majority of transplant centers, patients undergoing SLT must be less than 60 years of age. At those centers performing DLT or HLT, the usual age limit is between 50 and 55 years. Exceptions have been made in certain circumstances.

Patients with a history of systemic disease or prior malignancy are generally not considered as transplant candidates since they are at risk for more complications. Additionally, patients should not have evidence of renal or hepatic dysfunction since many of the immunosuppressive drugs used following transplantation can worsen the preexisting disease.

It is preferable to perform the transplant surgery on patients who have had no previous cardiothoracic surgery such as open lung biopsy, previous thoracotomy, or pneumothoraces requiring chemical or surgical pleurodesis. Previous surgery promotes scarring, adhesions, and fibrosis in the pleural space, which may make surgery technically

---

TABLE 4   Recipient Selection Criteria

Age <60 years (SLT)
Age <50–55 years (DLT, HLT)
Expected survival <18 months
No extrapulmonary or systemic disease*
No previous thoracic surgery*
No recent steroid use†
Adequate nutritional status
Adequate psychosocial status

---

* Relative contraindication.
† This criterion is controversial.

difficult. These problems are further exacerbated during HLT and some DLT procedures when the patient requires cardiopulmonary bypass with heparinization. Additionally, at those transplant centers that use the omental wrap anastomosis, previous abdominal surgery is a relative contraindication to transplantation since abdominal scar tissue may prevent mobilization of the omental pedicle.

A controversial issue in recipient selection has been the use of systemic corticosteroids prior to transplantation. Previously it was thought that steroids prior to transplantation might inhibit adequate healing of the anastomosis, the thoracotomy, or the sternotomy and thus increase the risk of anastomotic or surgical wound dehiscence. Therefore, at many transplant centers, patients have been required to discontinue steroids at least 1 month prior to transplantation. At our institution, patients have been transplanted successfully on doses ranging from 5 to 20 mg of prednisone per day without anastomotic or wound complications.[16] Recently five HLTs at the University Hospital in London, Ontario, were successfully performed with the patients on doses of prednisone ranging from 5 to 40 mg per day.[33]

A second controversy in recipient selection is the preoperative nutritional status of the patient. Due to the increased work of breathing required in patients with end-stage lung disease and the chronic infections in patients with CF, it is often difficult to maintain adequate nutritional status. Poor nutritional status results in difficulties with postoperative wound healing, can further compound complications related to drug-induced immunosuppression, and can preclude mobility following transplantation. Likewise, a patient undergoing transplantation who is significantly greater than his or her ideal body weight can develop postsurgical atelectasis and/or infections, resulting in a higher postoperative mortality. Therefore, the ideal transplant candidate should be within 10–15% of his or her ideal body weight.

A third controversial issue in lung transplant recipient selection is the ventilator-dependent patient. Ventilator-dependent patients are rapidly colonized by hospital flora soon after intubation and can become infected following transplantation once subjected to immunosuppression. In addition, the incidence of nosocomial infection in mechanically ventilated patients is significant. This should certainly be considered only a relative contraindication to transplantation since patients ventilated for short periods of time have undergone successful transplantation without postoperative infections.

Equally as important as the above medical recipient selec-

Poor nutritional status results in difficulties with postoperative wound healing, can further compound complications related to drug-induced immunosuppression, and can preclude mobility following transplantation.

Ventilator dependency should be considered only a relative contraindication to transplantation, since patients ventilated for short periods of time have been successfully transplanted without postoperative infection.

tion criteria are psychosocial selection criteria. Potential transplant candidates must have normal psychiatric evaluations and have a history of good medical compliance. They must be well motivated with a strong social support network. All patients should be nonsmokers for at least 1 year at the time of transplant evaluation. In addition, patients with a history of substance abuse should be excluded from transplant consideration.

CANDIDATE EVALUATION

Complete pulmonary function testing, including spirometry, lung volumes by body plethysmography, diffusion capacity, arterial blood gases, and, if tolerated, some form of exercise assessment, is performed.

After meeting the above recipient selection criteria, the patient undergoes an extensive pretransplant evaluation. The pretransplantation assessment includes the items listed in Table 5. Complete pulmonary function testing with spirometry, lung volumes by body plethysmography, diffusion capacity, arterial blood gases, and if tolerated, some form of exercise assessment is performed. At UTHSC-SA, the patient undergoes incremental cycle ergometer exercise testing as tolerated. At other institutions, a 6-minute walk or modified Bruce protocol is used to assess pretransplant exercise tolerance. Quantitative V/Q scans are performed to assess global lung function and to determine discrepancies between the lungs. Chest computed tomography is per-

---

TABLE 5   Candidate Evaluation

Pulmonary function testing
  Spirometry
  Lung volumes
  Diffusion capacity
  Arterial blood gases
  Exercise test (if tolerated)
Laboratory
  CBC
  SMA-20
  Urinalysis
  Creatinine clearance
Immunology
  Blood type
  HIV
  HbsAg
  VDRL
  Titers for CMV, EBV, VZV, HSV
  Skin tests: PPD and anergy panel
Quantitative V/Q scanning
Cardiac evaluation
  MUGA with RVEF and LVEF
  2-D echocardiogram, cardiac catheterization with coronary
    angiography
Chest CT
Consults from psychiatry and dental services

formed at some centers to look for possible bronchiectasis, which would preclude SLT, or to look for possible mass lesions not apparent on plain radiograph.

Preoperative cardiac evaluation includes an echocardiogram and radionuclide angiography with first pass to assess right and left ejection fractions. At many centers, patients undergo cardiac catheterization with coronary angiography. At UTHSC-SA, if pulmonary artery pressures are elevated at the time of the catheterization, then nitroprusside and oxygen are administered to assess reversibility of pulmonary hypertension. We have found that patients with reversible pulmonary hypertension have better postoperative pulmonary function and V/Q matching. At other transplant centers, the cardiac evaluation is conducted non-invasively and coronary angiography is performed only if clinically indicated.[7]

The majority of patients considered for transplantation have some component of right heart failure. This may vary from mild right heart failure in patients with obstructive lung disease to severe right heart failure, secondary to pulmonary pressures approaching that of the systemic circulation, in patients with PPH and end-stage restrictive lung disease. In general, SLT or DLT is arbitrarily performed on patients with right ventricular ejection fractions (RVEF) of higher than 25%. However, successful transplantation with RVEF lower than this have been reported. In addition, preliminary studies have shown marked improvement in post-transplant RVEF.[34]

Laboratory assessment should include a complete blood count (CBC), SMA-20, urinalysis, creatinine clearance, human immunodeficiency virus (HIV) testing, hepatitis serology, and titers for cytomegalovirus (CMV), Epstein-Barr virus (EBV), varicella zoster virus (VZV), and herpes simplex virus (HSV). Nutritional assessment is performed at some centers by obtaining total calorie counts and tricep skinfold measurements. Inpatient consultations from the psychiatric service and the dental service should be conducted on all patients. A PAP smear and a mammogram should be ordered on all female patients. On those patients with CF, ear, nose, and throat (ENT) evaluation with some form of sinus drainage procedure is indicated.

The role of preoperative rehabilitation training prior to transplantation is controversial. It is unclear in any patient population whether rehabilitation improves survival. Studies show that rehabilitation training does improve quality of life and exercise tolerance.[35] The majority of transplant programs do incorporate pretransplant rehabilitation. At some programs this is monitored by repeated 6-minute walks. At Toronto, patients undergoing pretransplant re-

*It is unclear in any patient population whether rehabilitation improves survival. Studies show, however, that rehabilitation training **does** improve quality of life and exercise tolerance.*

habilitation have improved 6-minute walk distances, from 57 m/min to 79 m/min.[7] At UTHSC-SA, preoperative reha-bilitation is not currently employed, and in fact several wheelchair-bound patients have undergone transplanta-tion with successful results.

At the Washington University Lung Transplant program, a recent analysis of 211 patients with end-stage pulmonary disease referred for transplantation was distributed as fol-lows: 52% of these patients had COPD, 18% had IPF, 9% had CF, and the remainder had other causes of pulmonary fibrosis or vascular disease. After meeting the recipient se-lection screening criteria, 46 of the referred patients were admitted for further inpatient evaluation and only 18 of these patients were accepted as potential transplant candi-dates. Of these 18 patients, 16 eventually received trans-plants and 2 died while awaiting their surgery.[36]

DONOR SELECTION

The criteria for pulmonary donation are shown in Table 6. The majority of potential donors are brain dead as a result of head trauma or a primary central nervous system event. The ideal donor should be less than 55–60 years of age. Serial chest radiographs should be grossly clear. When per-forming HLT or DLT, both lungs must meet radiologic crite-ria. However, when performing SLT, unilateral lung injury secondary to blunt or open trauma does not necessarily exclude the contralateral lung from consideration for trans-plantation.

The functional capacity of the potential donor lung is further assessed by gas exchange capability. A PaO_2 greater than 300 mmHg on an FIO_2 of 1.0 with a PEEP of 5 cmH_2O is preferred. Gas exchange not meeting these criteria may indicate potential V/Q problems. Other centers have used a PaO_2 greater than 100 mmHg on an FIO_2 of 0.4 for donor gas exchange criteria.

Since possible infectious agents can be transmitted by an infected donor organ, a Gram stain of a tracheal aspirate and/or a bronchoscopy is performed on all potential donor candidates. If organisms are present on the Gram stain with fewer than 10 epithelial cells and more than 25 white blood cells per high power field, the organs should not be consid-ered for donation. Additionally, if there is evidence of fun-gal elements on the Gram stain, the donor organs should be rejected. Many institutions perform bronchoscopy on the potential donor as part of the harvesting procedure.

TABLE 6   Donor Selection Criteria

Age <55 years
Normal chest radiograph
PaO_2 > 300 mmHg on FIO_2 of 1.0 and PEEP-5 cmH_2O
Normal sputum Gram stain and/or bronchoscopic exam
Negative HBsAg
Negative HIV

This is done to assess the presence of blood, purulence, or foreign bodies in the tracheobronchial tree not suggested by the chest radiograph or gross appearance of tracheal secretions. If the bronchoscopic examination is abnormal, the organs should be excluded from potential transplant donation.

Donor screening serologies, including HIV, hepatitis B, and CMV, complete the donor evaluation process. If hepatitis B surface antigen (HBsAg) or HIV antibody is present, the patient is not a donor candidate. As discussed for transplant recipients, lung harvesting is relatively contraindicated in donors with a history of previous thoracotomy because of pleural adhesions and resulting hemorrhagic complications.

Patients with hepatitis B surface antigen or HIV antibody are not suitable donor candidates.

DONOR–RECIPIENT COMPATIBILITY

When an acceptable donor organ becomes available for transplantation, certain donor–recipient compatibility must be met. Unlike other solid organ donations, SLT, HLT, and DLT are ABO matched only and not HLA matched. Lung graft preservation time is currently limited to 3 to 4 hours. This limited preservation time precludes HLA typing prior to transplantation.

Although not universal, most transplant centers perform donor and recipient CMV serology matching. A CMV-negative recipient receives organs only from a CMV-negative donor. A CMV-positive recipient can receive organs from a CMV-negative or -positive donor. There has been a mild increased incidence of post-transplant CMV pneumonia in CMV-negative patients who have received lungs from CMV-positive donors.

Donor–recipient size matching is assessed in various ways. At UTHSC-SA, the chest circumference of the transplant recipient is measured at the level of the nipple and matched to the corresponding donor chest wall circumference within 3 inches in either direction.[12] Other institutions have performed size matching by estimating chest wall size on a plain radiograph or by using a combination of body weight and chest wall circumference plus horizontal thoracic measurements.[7] Still other centers estimate the lung capacity of the donor using a height and sex nomogram and match this with that of the recipient.[37] Despite the method of size matching used, studies have shown that the donor lung soon approximates the recipient's lung capacity following transplantation.[37,38]

MONITORING FOLLOWING TRANSPLANTATION

Some transplant centers delay immunosuppressive therapy until the second or third postoperative day to optimize postoperative wound healing.

Immediately following transplantation, immunosuppressive therapy should be begun with corticosteroids, cyclosporin A, and azathioprine.[12] Previously at our center, all patients received postoperative cytolytic therapy with antilymphocyte globulin or the monoclonal T-cell inhibitor OKT3. Due to several outbreaks of CMV infection, empiric cytolytic therapy was discontinued.[39] At some transplant centers, immunosuppressive therapy is delayed until the second or third postoperative day to optimize postoperative wound healing.

How to best monitor the patient following transplantation to detect early rejection or infection remains controversial. Quantitative ventilation and perfusion to the lung graft was initially examined as an early indicator of graft rejection. In SLT recipients with emphysema and/or end-stage restrictive disease, early acute rejection was often heralded by a decrease in perfusion to the lung graft.[7] However, this was found to be neither sensitive nor specific for the diagnosis of rejection or infection. In fact, in those patients undergoing SLT for PPH, rejection is heralded by a decrease in ventilation to the lung graft and not a decrease in perfusion.[30]

The chest radiograph has been shown to be neither specific nor sensitive for early detection of infection or rejection.[40–42] In HLT recipients, rejection or infection in the first month following transplantation is associated with an abnormal chest radiograph in 74% of cases. However, after the first posttransplant month, the chest radiograph was found to be abnormal in only 23% of rejection episodes.[40]

Some centers have attempted to follow daily pulmonary function in order to detect early rejection or infection.[43,44] At these centers, patients are given home spirometers and instructed to document their FEV_1 (forced expiratory volume after 1 second) on a daily or twice-daily basis. Patients are told to notify the transplant center if the FEV_1 declines by more than 10%. Previous studies have attempted to correlate this decline in spirometry with findings on transbronchial biopsy. A study of 15 HLT patients in the United Kingdom showed a mean FEV_1 decrease of $10.4 \pm 6.9\%$ with biopsy-proven rejection and a mean FEV_1 decrease of $12.8 \pm 10.1\%$ with biopsy-proven infection.[44] The proponents of home spirometry suggest that monitoring of lung function enables early detection of acute episodes of rejection and/or infection and may be a useful indictor for obtaining transbronchial biopsies.[43]

A study of 34 HLT patients compared chest radiographs, pulmonary function, and results of transbronchial biopsy in acute lung infection and rejection. These investigators concluded that pulmonary function testing has an 86% sensitivity in detecting rejection in the first 3 months postoperatively, and decreases to 75% subsequently. For infection, the sensitivity is 75%. Pulmonary function testing could not distinguish between infection and rejection but had an 84% specificity for these two diagnoses combined. This study also concluded that the chest radiograph was sensitive early following transplantation but subsequently had only 19% specificity for rejection and 58% specificity for infection.[42] Thus although pulmonary function tests and chest radiographs have comparable sensitivities in the first 3 months following transplantation, the pulmonary function tests remain sensitive following this initial 3-month period, whereas chest radiographs may be normal. Spirometric measurements offer more sensitive monitoring of the lung graft and are a better guide of when to perform transbronchial biopsy than chest radiographs.

Many centers have performed surveillance transbronchial biopsies at various time periods following transplantation in order to detect asymptomatic rejection and/or infection. Initial proponents of HLT thought that monitoring the heart with routine endomyocardial biopsies, as is done for heart transplantation, would be a useful indicator for the rejection of the lungs as well. However, this was shown not to be the case, and either organ can reject separately.[45,46] Following this it was determined that transbronchial biopsy is useful in the detection of lung graft infection or rejection.[5,45–48] Higenbottam et al., evaluating the sensitivity and specificity of transbronchial biopsy for the diagnosis of rejection in HLT, have shown that transbronchial biopsy has an overall sensitivity of 84% and specificity of 100%.[48] In order to achieve these statistics, investigators have recommended that at least 18 transbronchial biopsies be performed from different lobes of the lung. It has been suggested that up to one third of lung rejection episodes may be missed if only four transbronchial specimens are taken.[49] A recent standardization of lung rejection by the Lung Rejection Study Group recommends a minimum of five transbronchial specimens be obtained in order to diagnose rejection.[50] Acute rejection is characterized pathologically by perivascular and interstitial mononuclear infiltrates. It is important to remember that CMV infection is also associated with perivascular lymphocytic infiltrates and often poses a problem for the pathologist in differentiating rejection from infection.

Transbronchial biopsy is useful in the detection of lung graft infection or rejection.

It has been suggested that up to one third of lung rejection episodes may be missed if only four transbronchial specimens are taken.

Another less invasive technique for monitoring graft function is bronchoalveolar lavage (BAL). Some studies have shown that the finding of donor specific alloreactivity in BAL lymphocytes may be a sensitive marker of lung allograft rejection, at least in HLT recipients.[51] Preliminary studies in SLT and DLT recipients do not support the sensitivity of the BAL-primed lymphocyte test for the detection of acute lung rejection.[52] In addition, in SLT and DLT recipients, the BAL cell profile analysis could not distinguish between CMV pneumonia or rejection.[52,53]

At UTHSC-SA patients are followed on a weekly basis in the outpatient transplant clinic for the first 6 weeks following transplantation. At each visit the patient is evaluated by one of the pulmonary transplant physicians. Weekly studies include a CBC in order to monitor the white blood cell count on azathioprine, a SMA-20 to follow liver function tests and creatinine on azathioprine and cyclosporin, a chest radiograph, routine spirometry, and constant workload cycle oximetry. If there is a change in clinical symptoms reported by the patient, a new infiltrate on the chest radiograph, a reduction in spirometry of more than 10%, or desaturation on exercise oximetry of more than 4–5%, transbronchial biopsy is performed. At UTHSC-SA, bronchoscopies are not performed unless one of the above indications is met. Although surveillance bronchoscopies have been recommended for detection of asymptomatic rejection, no randomized studies have been undertaken to determine differences in outcome between treatment and nontreatment in patients with asymptomatic rejection diagnosed by transbronchial biopsy.

RESULTS

Emphysema

As previously stated, emphysema was initially considered to be a contraindication to SLT. Since 1989, approximately 100 SLTs for end-stage obstructive lung disease have been performed in the world. Currently, obstructive pulmonary disease accounts for over 50% of referrals to large transplant centers.[36]

At UTHSC-SA, 25 SLTs have been performed on 24 patients with obstructive lung disease with 1- and 2-year actuarial survival rates of 75.87% and 70.03%. Underlying diseases in these patients include 11 patients with panlobular emphysema secondary to α_1-ATD and 12 patients with centrilobular emphysema secondary to tobacco use. In addition, one patient underwent SLT for end-stage obstructive lung disease due to bronchiolitis obliterans.

Figure 6 shows posteroanterior chest radiographs of a 40-year-old man with α_1-ATD before and after right SLT. A postoperative quantitative V/Q scan from the same patient is shown in Figure 7, revealing the majority of ventilation and perfusion going to the transplanted right lung.

The functional results in 12 patients who have survived at least 1 year following SLT are shown in Table 7. This table shows results of pulmonary function testing preoperatively, 3 months, 6 months, and 12 months post-SLT, and results of symptom-limited, graded-cycle exercise testing and quantitative V/Q lung scans at 3 months, 6 months, and 12 months post-SLT. From these data, the following conclusions can be made. SLT markedly improves lung function by 3 months postsurgery in patients with end-stage obstructive lung disease and this improvement is sustained for at least 12 months following transplantation. At 1 year post-transplant, these patients continued to show no evidence of ventilatory limitation to exercise as evidenced by stable saturations during exercise and an adequate ventilatory reserve. In addition, the majority of ventilation and perfusion goes to the lung graft following transplantation. Further analysis of these data show no difference in the above parameters between α_1-ATD patients and patients with COPD secondary to tobacco use.[54] As stated previously, no difference was observed between those patients undergoing right versus left graft placement.[15]

In the United Kingdom at the National Heart and Lung Institute, 25 patients with end-stage obstructive airways disease underwent SLT between March 1988 and August 1990.[55] These 25 patients constituted 40% of all of the SLTs performed at that center during this period. Nineteen of these patients had bilateral emphysema, secondary to α_1-ATD in 12 and secondary to tobacco use in 7. Six patients were women with lymphangiomyomatosis. In this group of patients, the actuarial survival was 92% at 1 month and 78% at 1 year. All patients had marked improvement in their symptoms, improving from NYHA Class III/IV to NYHA Class I or II. There was significant improvement in spirometry from a preoperative FEV_1 of $21 \pm 9\%$ of predicted to a postoperative FEV_1 of $40 \pm 13\%$ of predicted at 3 months following transplantation and $47 \pm 16\%$ of predicted at 1 year following transplantation. Quantitative V/Q lung scans indicated that approximately 80% of both ventilation and perfusion were distributed to the transplanted lung.

At the University of Toronto, DLT has been performed for the treatment of end-stage emphysema. Initially, six patients with nonseptic obstructive airways disease under-

SLT markedly improves lung function by 3 months after surgery in patients with end-stage obstructive lung disease; this improvement is sustained for at least 12 months following transplantation.

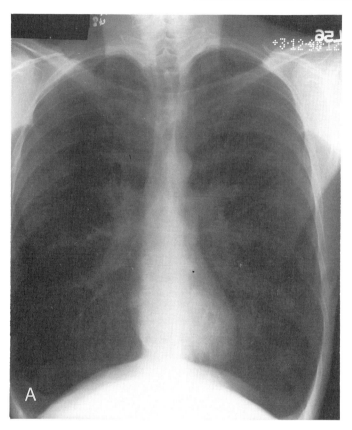

FIG. 6   (A) Posteroanterior radiograph before right-sided SLT for α_1-antitrypsin deficiency. (*Figure continues*)

TABLE 7   Functional Results at 1 Year Following SLT for Obstructive Disease

	FEV$_1$ (%)	FVC (%)	FEV$_1$/FVC	TLC (%)	DL$_{CO}$ (%)
Pre	15 ± 4	47 ± 7	.25 ± .04	154 ± 34	22 ± 11
3 mo post	54 ± 9	56 ± 6	.76 ± .09	123 ± 14	75 ± 13
6 mo post	59 ± 12	62 ± 9	.72 ± .08	113 ± 7	72 ± 11
12 mo post	59 ± 12	63 ± 8	.72 ± .10	120 ± 12	76 ± 14

	VE$_{max}$ (% MVV)	SaO$_{2max}$ (%)	V (% to SLT)	Q
3 mo post	55 ± 18	94 ± 3	86 ± 10	86 ± 8
6 mo post	67 ± 20	95 ± 4	83 ± 11	75 ± 6
12 mo post	65 ± 17	95 ± 3	88 ± 4	79 ± 8

FEV$_1$, Forced expiratory volume in 1 second; FVC, forced vital capacity; FEV$_1$/FVC, ratio of FEV$_1$ to FVC; TLC, total lung capacity; DL$_{CO}$, diffusing capacity; VE$_{max}$, minute ventilation at maximum exercise; SaO$_{2max}$, arterial oxygen saturation; V, ventilation; Q, perfusion.

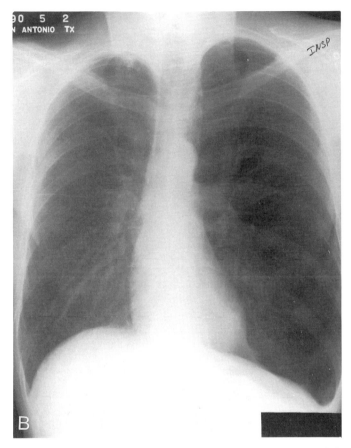

FIG. 6 (*continued*) (B) Posteroanterior radiograph after right-sided SLT for α_1-antitrypsin deficiency.

went DLT: three patients had α_1-ATD, one patient had OB, one patient had centrilobular emphysema secondary to tobacco use, and one patient had eosinophilic granuloma. All patients underwent en bloc DLT with three end-to-end anastomoses. All six recipients were alive and well 5–15 months following transplantation at the time of the report,[29] and all recipients had achieved a normal level of function. Ischemic airway complications occurred in three of the six DLT recipients.

A second report from the Minneapolis Heart Institute described six patients with end-stage emphysema subjected to DLT. Five of these patients had α_1-ATD and one patient had obstructive lung disease secondary to chemical inhalation. In this group of patients, two developed acute rejection responding to methylprednisolone bolus and four developed CMV infections of which three were treated successfully and one succumbed. Of the five surviving patients, three patients returned to work, one patient was in

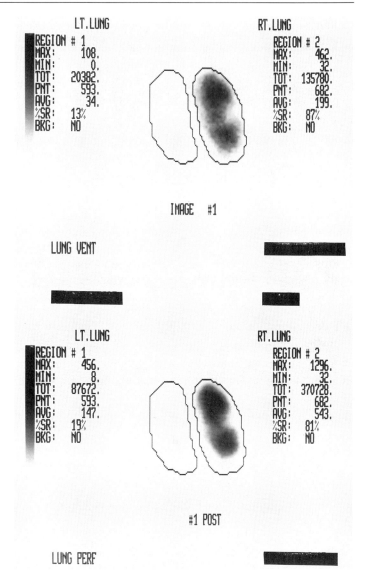

FIG. 7 A posterior view of a postoperative quantitative V/Q scan on the patient described in Figure 6.

an active rehabilitation program, and one was at home.[56] All patients showed significant improvement and near normalization of their pulmonary function by 6 months following surgery.

A third option for the treatment of emphysema is HLT. Seventeen emphysematous patients underwent HLT at the National Heart and Lung Institute in London. Eleven of these patients were followed up for a minimum of 1 year. Seven of these patients had α_1-ATD. In this group of patients, the actuarial 1-year survival was 91% and the 2-year survival was 76%.[57] All survivors achieved an excellent functional level.

Many of the above-cited studies report good functional results following SLT, DLT, or HLT for nonseptic obstructive lung disease. A recent study compared outcomes in SLT recipients to those in DLT recipients for obstructive lung disease. There was no difference in the preoperative values for pulmonary function tests, arterial blood gases, quantitative V/Q lung scans, or 6-minute walk tests. Following transplantation, DLT recipients had a higher FEV_1 and a higher forced vital capacity than SLT recipients. However, the $FEV_1\%$ was not different between the two groups. Arterial blood gas analyses were also not different between the two groups. The results of 3-month postoperative 6-minute walk distances were markedly improved in both groups and comparable following transplantation.[58] No study has compared results of all three procedures (SLT, HLT, and DLT) for the treatment of obstructive disease.

This leaves the transplant physician with several options. SLT does serve a number of advantages over DLT or HLT in obstructive lung disease patients. In all forms of cardiopulmonary transplantation, the controlling factor is the limited donor organ supply. If SLT is used, three recipients (i.e., two SLTs and one heart) may be able to benefit from the donor organs. SLT is a technically simpler surgery than either DLT or HLT and cardiopulmonary bypass can usually be avoided. Furthermore, it remains to be seen if the incidence of chronic rejection (i.e., OB) is the same following each of these three surgical techniques.

In patients undergoing transplantation for emphysema due to α_1-ATD, concerns have been raised regarding postoperative α_1-antitrypsin substitution. Transplantation for α_1-ATD is a relatively recent technique, and the long-term results remain to be seen. To date, it appears that α_1-antitrypsin repletion is not necessary. If lung injury in allografts placed in α_1-ATD recipients does not occur any more rapidly than it does in other α_1-ATD patients then emphysema would require 40 years to develop and there is no need for enzyme replacement.

SLT has a number of advantages over DLT or HLT in obstructive lung disease patients.

Cystic Fibrosis

Cystic fibrosis is the most common, lethal genetic abnormality in the Caucasian population. It is an autosomal recessive trait affecting 1 out 2,000 live births in North America. CF is characterized by a generalized epithelial dysfunction in numerous organs, particularly the lungs, the pancreas, the skin, and the gastrointestinal tract. Many unique concerns arise when considering the possibility of transplantation in patients with CF. CF is a multiorgan disease, and it is unclear whether lung transplantation will result in improved long-term survival. Secondly, these patients are prone to chronic pulmonary infections, which raises the concern that infections could recur following transplantation once subjected to immunosuppression. Finally, questions have arisen as to whether the CF pathophysiology could develop in the transplanted lungs.

In 1983, the first patient with CF underwent transplantation at the University of Pittsburgh. A HLT was performed.[59] Since this time, numerous HLTs have been performed for CF. In the past 5 years, approximately 90 patients have undergone HLT for CF in the United Kingdom.[60] The approximate waiting time for HLT is 7 months and it is estimated that up to one third of patients die while awaiting HLT.[60] An additional 30 HLTs for CF have been performed in Europe, and approximately 33 HLTs for CF have been performed in North America. Recently, the University of Toronto has performed DLT for the treatment of CF.[61]

At the Hospital for Sick Children and Papworth Hospital in the United Kingdom, 112 patients with CF were referred for HLT over a 4.5-year period and 83 were accepted. Of these 83, 26 died while awaiting HLT and 32 underwent transplantation. The cumulative survival in this group of 32 patients was 72.29% at 1 year and 55.59% at 3 years. This is comparable to survivor results in HLT recipients without CF. The mortality rate was slightly higher in the CF group during the first year after transplantation but was lower than other HLT recipients at 3 years. In multicenter combined statistics, actuarial survival rates in HLT performed for CF vary between 66 and 78% at 1 year, 70 and 72% at 2 years, 55 and 72% at 3 years, and 60% at 4 years. Again, this is similar to actuarial statistics obtained in HLT recipients with other underlying diseases.

At what point should a patient with CF be referred for transplantation? Pulmonary indicators of poor survival (i.e., less than 2 years) include FEV_1 less than 25–30% of predicted, hypoxic and/or hypercapnic respiratory failure, the development of right heart failure, and the minimum arterial oxygen saturation during a 12-minute walk.[60] Additionally, poor nutritional status is an indicator of poor survival. CF patients meeting any of these above specific criteria should be referred for transplantation.

There are several unique problems involved with recipient screening in patients with CF that deserve mention. This group of patients may have had a history of spontaneous pneumothorax requiring pleurodesis, which is a relative contraindication to transplantation. In addition, CF patients are prone to the development of lung cavitation and subsequent mycetoma formation, which is also a relative contraindication to transplantation. Resistant bacterial infections, common in CF patients, also may exclude a patient from potential transplantation. It is not uncommon to see evidence of portal hypertension and cirrhosis in CF patients, which is an absolute contraindication to transplantation although some consideration has been given to performing HLT or DLT and liver transplantation concurrently.[60]

Due to the frequent finding of sinusitis in CF patients, many transplant centers perform a Caldwell-Luc procedure with nasal antrostomies preoperatively to prevent postoperative sinus drainage from infecting the transplanted grafts. Some programs have performed an alternative procedure of preoperative transnasal antrostomy and endoscopic ethmoidectomy. Still other centers treat symptoms of bronchitis and sinusitis with standard courses of oral or parenteral antibiotics only, prior to transplantation.[62]

Performing transplantation in CF patients may result in several technical problems intraoperatively. Hemorrhage secondary to pleural adhesions may result. Additionally, CF patients tend to have highly vascularized mediastinal nodes that may require extensive dissection. Some of these hemorrhagic problems have been alleviated by the perioperative use of aprotinin (Trasylol).[63] In an attempt to reduce postoperative infection, both the recipient and donor tracheal stumps may be washed with Betadine in the operating room before performing the anastomosis, although this has not been proven beneficial.

Postoperatively in CF patients, most centers administer antibiotic prophylaxis, usually with a third-generation cephalosporin and flucloxacillin for 48 hours pending donor and recipient culture results. Following transplantation, the morbidity of distal intestinal obstruction syndrome (the adult equivalent of meconium ileus) and pancreatitis can be diminished by routine postoperative administration of N-acetylcysteine and lactulose. Pancreatic enzymes should be administered to ensure absorption.

Several unique problems related to immunosuppression have arisen. Early on, it was apparent that CF patients may require 5–10 times the total daily dose of cyclosporin A than other transplant recipients. This may be due to altered cyclosporin pharmacokinetics or absorption problems unique to CF patients. In order to reduce the total daily dose and cost by up to one third of that used previously,[64] it is recommended that cyclosporin A be administered three or four times per day in this patient population. It is also

Resistant bacterial infections, common in CF patients, may preclude transplantation.

Due to the frequent finding of sinusitis in CF patients, many transplant centers perform a preoperative Caldwell-Luc procedure with nasal antrostomies to prevent postoperative sinus drainage from infecting the transplanted grafts.

important to monitor patients blood glucoses carefully as CF patients have been reported to have an increased incidence of diabetes mellitus triggered by corticosteroids.[65]

The incidence of infection and rejection in HLT recipients with CF is not statistically different from the incidence of infection and rejection in other HLT recipients.[65] Transbronchial biopsy is used to follow these patients posttransplant.[66] Both surveillance bronchoscopy as well as symptom-indicated bronchoscopy suggested by new radiographic infiltrate, worsening clinical symptoms, or a decrease in $FEV_1\%$ have been performed.[66] In adults, flexible fiberoptic bronchoscopy is performed, whereas in children who require less than a 7 mm French endotracheal tube intraoperatively, rigid bronchoscopy is the bronchoscopic procedure of choice. For the diagnosis of rejection, the sensitivities and specificities of these procedures are 91% and 69%, respectively, in this patient population.[66]

Pulmonary function following HLT for CF has typically normalized by 3 months postoperatively and remains stable at 80% of the predicted values from 3 months onward. In the first 28 patients undergoing HLT at Papworth, the mean FEV_1 improved from 19% of predicted pre-HLT to 81% of predicted by 3 months post-HLT. It is certainly clear that the quality of life improves following HLT for CF.[67] Finally, it has been shown that within the 10% confidence level, HLT improves the chance of survival in patients with CF.[60,67]

To date, bronchiectasis has not developed in the transplanted organs. At least up until 3 years post-HLT, the characteristic bioelectric mucosal potential abnormality found in the respiratory mucosa in CF has not recurred in the transplanted lungs. Studies examining this electropotential difference have shown that although the donor lungs do not acquire the electrochemical defect associated with CF, the defect does remain above the tracheal anastomosis.[68,69] Furthermore, the airway infections typical of CF have not recurred in the majority of transplant recipients.

PROBLEMS IN TRANSPLANTATION

Two of the many problems facing lung transplantation are graft rejection and CMV infection.

Rejection

Chronic rejection or OB initially developed in 50% of patients within 2–35 months following HLT.[20] However, with augmentation of post-transplant immunosuppression using a three-drug regimen, OB can at least be arrested[23] and perhaps the incidence can be decreased to 20–30%.[23,24]

Clinically, OB presents with progressive dyspnea on exertion. Spirometry typically reveals an obstructive ventilatory defect.[70] Serial maximum expiratory flow volume loops in HLT recipients with OB reveal dynamic airway compression in the trachea over most of the vital capacity and subsequent shortening of the flow plateau indicating a progressively earlier shift of the site of flow limitation from extrapulmonary to intrapulmonary airways.

The etiology of OB remains unclear. There are several theories proposed in the literature. Preoperative seropositive status for CMV, postoperative CMV infection, and organ grafts from seropositive donors appear to increase the incidence of OB.[71] It is unclear if CMV is a direct etiologic factor or if CMV infection increases the incidence of recurrent acute infection, which in turn increases the incidence of OB. Others believe that OB results from undetected, asymptomatic, untreated rejection.[72] Proponents of undiagnosed rejection leading to OB recommend surveillance transbronchial biopsies to detect and treat early rejection.[24,72,73] Others have recommended surveillance BAL to look for a positive primed lymphocyte test correlating with OB.[74]

The etiology of OB remains unclear.

Chest radiographic findings in OB are nonspecific and include decreased peripheral vascular markings, slight volume loss, subsegmental atelectasis, and irregular areas of increased opacity. High resolution computed tomography has also been found to be nonspecific and may detect mild peripheral bronchiectasis and/or decreased peripheral vascular markings. Radiography is certainly not a useful way to survey for OB.[75]

Initially it appeared that the incidence of OB in SLT or DLT was less than the 25–50% reported with HLT. Now that SLT and DLT recipients have been followed for a time period comparable to HLT recipients, it is apparent that this initial conclusion was incorrect. A 1989 report described an SLT recipient who developed OB 4 months following transplantation.[28] A second case report described an SLT recipient who developed OB 9 months following transplantation. The patient progressively deteriorated and eventually died 21 months post-transplant.[27] A comparative study of DLT versus HLT recipients reported a 54% incidence of OB in HLT recipients and a 62% incidence of OB in DLT recipients.[26] The Toronto Lung Transplant Group, in contrast, has documented a 19% incidence of OB in SLT and a 12% incidence in DLT recipients.[76] Currently it appears that there is probably a similar incidence of OB in all three forms of transplantation.[25,26]

Cytomegalovirus Infection

Cytomegalovirus is another major problem facing the field of lung transplantation. At UTHSC-SA, CMV has been a primary cause of morbidity and mortality. In the first 31 SLT recipients at our center, 22 received cytolytic therapy postoperatively, including ALG or OKT3. Nine subsequent patients did not receive cytolytic therapy. In these patients, 17 of the 22 receiving cytolytic therapy developed CMV infection, whereas only 3 of 9 who did not receive cytolytic therapy developed CMV infection. Cytolytic therapy appeared to increase the incidence of postoperative infection with CMV and should not be used routinely in lung transplant patients.[39] As stated previously, CMV may lead to an increased incidence of OB.[71] Some centers have advocated donor recipient matching of CMV status. In other words, CMV antibody-negative recipients should only receive organs from CMV antibody-negative donors.[77] In one study of 18 patients who were preoperatively CMV negative, 8 received CMV-positive organ donation. Five of these eight developed CMV pneumonia, and this proved fatal in three of these patients. In contrast, only 3 of 10 antibody-negative patients who received antibody-negative organ donation developed CMV infection. One of these patients died.[77] Currently, it does appear that ganciclovir treatment is effective for the treatment of symptomatic CMV infections in lung transplant recipients.[78,79]

CONCLUSION

There are numerous other problems facing the field of lung transplantation that are beyond the scope of this chapter. Perhaps the largest problem is the shortage of donor organs. As of August 1991, there were 551 patients awaiting lung transplantation in the United States alone.[80] Advancement in the areas of organ preservation and donor recruitment may alleviate this shortage in the future.

SLT, DLT, and HLT appear to be promising treatments for patients with end-stage lung disease. Strategies for lung transplantation are constantly evolving and what is currently considered standard practice is certain to change in the future. Clearly, the next decade will yield vast advances in the field of lung transplantation.

References

1. Reitz BA, Wallwork J, Hunt SA et al: Heart-lung transplantation: successful therapy for patients with pulmoanry vascular disease. N Engl J Med 306:557, 1982

2. Toronto Lung Transplant Group: Unilateral lung transplantation for pulmonary fibrosis. N Engl J Med 314:1140, 1986

3. Hardy JD, Webb WR, Dalton ML, Walker GR: Lung homotransplantation in man. JAMA 186:1065, 1963

4. Veith FJ, Kamholz SL, Mollenkopf FB, Montefusco CM: Lung transplantation 1983. Transplantation 35(4):271, 1983

5. McCarthy PM: Outcome improving for lung transplant patients. Cleve Clin J Med 57(8):673, 1990

6. Grossman RF, Frost A, Zamel N et al: Results of single-lung transplantation for bilateral pulmonary fibrosis. N Engl J Med 322:727, 1990

7. The Toronto Lung Transplant Group: Experience with single-lung transplantation for pulmonary fibrosis. JAMA 259(15):2258, 1988

8. Veith FJ, Koerner SK, Siegelman SS et al: Single lung transplantation in experimental and human emphysema. Ann Surg 178(4):463, 1973

9. Stevens PM, Johnson PC, Bell RL et al: Regional ventilation and perfusion after lung transplantation in patients with emphysema. N Engl J Med 282(5):245, 1970

10. Veith FJ, Koerner SK, Attai LA et al: Single-lung transplantation in emphysema. Lancet May 27:1138, 1972

11. Mal H, Andreassian B, Pamela F et al: Unilateral lung transplantation in end-stage pulmonary emphysema. Am Rev Respir Dis 140:797, 1989

12. Calhoon JH, Grover FL, Gibbons WJ et al: Single lung transplantation—alternative indications and technique. J Thorac Cardiovasc Surg 101(5):816, 1991

13. Trulock EP, Egan TM, Kouchoukos NT et al: Single lung transplantation for severe chronic obstructive pulmonary disease. Chest 96(4):738, 1989

14. Levine SM, Gibbons WJ, Bryan CL et al: Single lung transplantation for primary pulmonary hypertension. Chest 98:1107, 1990

15. Levine SM, Gibbons WJ, Bryan CL et al: Effect of graft position on pulmonary function after single lung transplantation for chronic obstructive lung disease. Chest 98(2):7S, 1990 (Abstract)

16. Bryan CL, Anzueto A, Levine SM et al: Corticosteroid therapy does not potentiate bronchial anastomotic complications in single lung transplantation (SLT) (Abstract). Am Rev Respir Dis 143(4):A461, 1991

17. Cooley DA, Bloodwell RD, Hallman GL et al: Organ transplantation for advanced cardiopulmonary disease. Ann Thorac Surg 8:300, 1969

18. Lillehei CW: Discussion of Wildevuur CRH, Benfield JR. A review of 23 human lung transplantations by 20 surgeons. Ann Thorac Surg 9:489, 1970

19. Losman JG, Campbell CD, Replogle RL, Barnard CN: Joint transplantation of the heart and lungs. Past experience and present potentials. J Cardiovasc Surg 23:440, 1982

20. Burke CM, Theordore J, Baldwin JC et al: Twenty-eight cases of human heart-lung transplantation. Lancet March 8:517, 1986

21. Reichart B, Reichenspurner H, Meiser B: Heart-lung transplantation in 1990—Indications, surgical technique, postoperative complications and outcome. Thorac Cardiovasc Surg 38:271, 1990

22. Kelpetko W, Wollenek G, Laczkovics A et al: Domino transplantation of heart-lung and heart: an approach to overcome the scarcity of donor organs. J Heart Lung Transplant 10:129, 1991

23. Glanville AR, Baldwin JC, Burke CM et al: Obliterative bronchiolitis after heart-lung transplantation: apparent arrest by augmented immunosuppression. Ann Intern Med 107:300, 1987

24. McCarthy PM, Starnes VA, Theodore J et al: Improved survival after heart-lung transplantation. J Thorac Cardiovasc Surg 99:54, 1990

25. Maurer JR, Morrison D, Winton TL, Patterson GA: Late pulmonary complications of isolated lung transplantation. Transplant Proc 23(1):1224, 1991

26. Kennan RJ, Bruzzone P, Paradis IL et al: Similarity of pulmonary rejection patterns among heart-lung and double-lung transplant recipients. Transplantation 51(1):176, 1991

27. LoCicero J, Robinson PG, Fisher M: Chronic rejection in single-lung transplantation manifested by obliterative bronchiolitis. J Thorac Cardiovasc Surg 99:1059, 1990

28. McGregor CGA, Dark JH, Hilton CJ et al: Early results of single lung transplantation in patients with end-stage pulmonary fibrosis. J Thorac Cardiovasc Surg 98:350, 1989

29. Cooper JD, Patterson GA, Grossman R, et al: Double-lung transplant for advanced chronic obstructive lung disease. Am Rev Respir Dis 139:303, 1989

30. Levine SM, Jenkinson SG, Bryan CL et al: Ventilation perfusion inequalities during graft rejection in patients undergoing single lung transplantation for primary pulmonary hypertension. Chest (In press)

31. Patterson GA, Todd TR, Cooper JD et al: Airway complications after double lung transplantation. J Thorac Cardiovasc Surg 99:14, 1990

32. Noirclere J, Metras D, Vaillant A et al: Bilateral bronchial anastomosis in double lung and heart-lung transplantation. Eur J Cardio Thorac Surg 4:314, 1990

33. Novick RJ, Menkis AH, McKenzie FN et al: The safety of low-dose prednisone before and immediately after heart-lung transplantation. Ann Thorac Surg 51:642, 1991

34. Yeog TK, Kramer MR, Marshall S et al: Changes in cardiac morphology and function following single-lung transplantation. Transplant Proc 23(1):1226, 1991

35. Belman MJ, Mittman C: Ventilatory muscle training improves exercise capacity in chronic obstructive pulmonary disease patients. Am Rev Respir Dis 121:273, 1980

36. Egan TM, Trulock EP, Boychuk J et al: Analysis of referrals for lung transplantation. Chest 99:867, 1991

37. Otulana BA, Mist BA, Scott JP et al: The effect of recipient lung size on lung physiology after heart-lung transplantation. Transplantation 48(4):625, 1989

38. Lloyd KS, Holland VA, Noon GP, Lawrence EC: Pulmonary function after heart-lung transplantation using larger donor organs. Am Rev Respir Dis 142:1026, 1990

39. Calhoon JH, Nichols L, Davis R et al: Single lung transplantation—factors in postoperative cytomegalovirus infection. J Thorac Cardiovasc Surg (In Press)

40. Millet B, Higenbottam TW, Flower CDR et al: The radiographic appearances of infection and acute rejection of the lung after heart-lung transplantation. Am Rev Respir Dis 140:62, 1989

41. Herman SJ, Rappaport DC, Weisbrod GL et al: Single-lung transplantation: imaging features. Radiology 170:89, 1989

42. Otulana BA, Higenbottam T, Scott J et al: Lung function associated with histologically diagnosed acute lung rejection and pulmonary infection in heart-lung transplant patients. Am Rev Respir Dis 14:329, 1990

43. Otulana BA, Higenbottam TW, Scott JP et al: Pulmonary function monitoring allows diagnosis of rejection in heart-lung transplant recipients. Transplant Proc 21(1):2583, 1989

44. Otulana BA, Higenbottam T, Ferrari L et al: The use of home spirometry in detecting acute lung rejection and infection following heart-lung transplantation. Chest 97(2):353, 1990

45. Sleiman C, Groussard O, Mal H et al: Clinical use of transbronchial biopsy in single-lung transplantation. Transplantation 51(4):927, 1991

46. Starnes VA, Theodore J, Oyer PE et al: Pulmonary infiltrates after heart-lung transplantation: evaluation by serial transbronchial biopsies. J Thorac Cardiovasc Surg 98:945, 1989

47. Starnes VA, Theodore J, Oyer PE et al: Evaluation of heart-lung transplant recipients with prospective, serial transbronchial biopsies and pulmonary function studies. J Thorac Cardiovasc Surg 98:683, 1989

48. Higenbottam T, Stewart S, Penketh A, Wallwork J: Transbronchial lung biopsy for the diagnosis of rejection in heart-lung transplant patients. Transplantation 46:532, 1988

49. Scott JP, Smyth RL, Higenbottam T et al: Transbronchial biopsy after lung transplantation. J Thorac Cardiovasc Surg 101:935, 1991

50. Yousem SA, Berry GJ, Brunt EM et al: A working formulation for the standardization of nomenclature in the diagnosis of heart and lung rejection: Lung rejection study group. J Heart Transplant 9(6):593, 1990

51. Rabinowich H, Zeevi A, Paradis IL et al: Proliferative responses of bronchoalveolar lavage lymphocytes from heart-lung transplant patients. Transplantation 49:115, 1990

52. Ettinger NA, Tsugi H, Muthuplackal J et al: The use of bronchoalveolar lavage to distinguish infection from rejection in single and double lung transplantation (Abstract). Am Rev Respir Dis 143:A600, 1991

53. Shennib H, Nguyen D: Bronchoalveolar lavage in lung transplantation. Ann Thorac Surg 51:335, 1991

54. Anzueto A, Levine SM, Bryan CL et al: Pulmonary function and exercise breathing patterns after single lung transplantation for chronic obstructive lung disease and alpha-1-antitrypsin deficiency (Abstract). Am Rev Respir Dis 143(4):A460, 1991

55. Yacoub M, Khaghani A, Theodoropoulos S et al: Single-lung transplantation for obstructive airway disease. Transplant Proc 23(1):1213, 1991

56. Emery RW, Graif JL, Hale K et al: Treatment of end-stage chronic obstructive pulmonary disease with double lung transplantation. Chest 99(3):533, 1991

57. Khaghani A, Banner N, Ozdogan E et al: Medium-term results of combined heart and lung transplantation for emphysema. J Heart Lung Transplant 10:15, 1991

58. Patterson GA, Maurer JR, Williams TJ et al: Comparison of outcomes of double and single lung transplantation for obstructive lung disease. J Thorac Cardiovasc Surg 101:623, 1991

59. Gallagher SL, Lawrence PA: Heart-lung transplantation: the patient with cystic fibrosis. Crit Care Nurs Q 13(4):32, 1991

60. Higenbottam TW, Whitehead B: Heart-lung transplantation for cystic fibrosis. J R Soc Med 84(18), 1991

61. Patterson GA, Cooper JD, Goldman B et al: Technique of successful double-lung transplantation. Ann Thorac Surg 1988; 45:626, 1988

62. Lewiston N, King V, Umetsu D et al: Cystic fibrosis patients who have undergone heart-lung transplantation benefit from maxillary sinus antrostomy and repeated sinus lavage. Transplant Proc 23(1):1207, 1991

63. Bidstrup BP, Royston D, Sapsford RN, Taylor KM: Reduction in blood loss and blood use after cardiopulmonary bypass with high dose aprotinin (Trasylol). J Thorac Cardiovasc Surg 97:364, 1989

64. Scott JP, Smyth RL, Higgenbottam TW et al: Cyclosporine dosing in cystic fibrosis after transplantation. Transplantation 48:544, 1989

65. Heart and lung transplantation for terminal cystic fibrosis. J Thorac Cardiovasc Surg 101:633, 1991

66. Scott JP, Higenbottam TW, Smyth RL et al: Transbronchial biopsies in children after heart-lung transplantation. Pediatrics 86:698, 1990

67. Caine N, Sharples LD, Smyth R et al: Survival and quality of life of cystic fibrosis patients before and after heart-lung transplantation. Transplant Proc 23(1):1203, 1991

68. Alton EWFW, Khagani A, Taylor RFH et al: Effect of heart-lung transplantation on airway potential difference in patients with and without cystic fibrosis. Eur Respir J 4:5, 1991

69. Wood A, Higenbottam T, Jackson M et al: Airway mucosal bioelectric potential difference in cystic fibrosis after lung transplantation. Am Rev Respir Dis 140:1645, 1989

70. Estenne M, Ketelbant P, Primo G, Yernault JC: Human heart-lung transplantation: Physiologic aspects of the denervated lung and post-transplant obliterative bronchiolitis. Am Rev Respir Dis 135:976, 1987

71. Kennan RJ, Lega ME, Dummer JS et al: Cytomegalovirus seriologic status and postoperative infection correlated with risk of developing chronic rejection after pulmonary transplantation. Transplantation 51(2):433, 1991

72. Scott JP, Higenbottam TW, Sharples L et al: Risk factors for obliterative bronchiolitis in heart-lung transplant recipients. Transplantation 51(4):813, 1991

73. Burdine J, Hertz MI, Snover DC, Bolman RM III: Heart-lung and lung transplantation: Perioperative pulmonary dysfunction. Transplant Proc 23(1):1176, 1991

74. Griffith BP, Paradis IL, Zeevi A et al: Immunologically mediated disease of the airways after pulmonary transplantation. Ann Surg 208(3):371, 1988

75. Morrish WF, Herman SJ, Weisbrod GL et al: Bronchiolitis obliterans after lung transplantation: findings at chest radiography and high-resolution CT. Radiology 179:487, 1991

76. Williams TJ, Grossman RF, Maurer JR: Long-term functional follow-up of lung transplant recipients. Clin Chest Med 11:347, 1990

77. Hutter JA, Scott J, Wreghitt T et al: The importance of cytomegalovirus in heart-lung transplant recipients. Chest 95(3):627, 1989

78. Steinhoff G, Behrend M, Wagner TOF et al: Early diagnosis and effective treatment of pulmonary CMV infection after lung transplantation. J Heart Lung Transplant 10:9, 1991

79. Cerrina J, Bavoux E, Ladurie FL et al: Ganciclovir treatment of cytomegalovirus infection in heart-lung and double-lung transplant recipients. Transplant Proc 23(1):1174, 1991

80. Update from the United Network for Organ Sharing: 7(9):1, Sept. 1991

CYSTIC FIBROSIS

CYNTHIA A. ZAMORA, MD
ANTONIO ANZUETO, MD

Cystic fibrosis (CF) is the most common lethal genetic disease in the Caucasian population. The condition is transmitted as an autosomal recessive trait and occurs in 1 of every 1,500–2,500 live births in whites. The incidence of CF in other ethnic populations, including American blacks and Orientals, is 1 in every 17,000–70,000 live births.[1] A major gene defect (ΔF508) responsible for 68% of the gene mutations associated with this illness has recently been identified.[2–4] Carriers of the CF gene are asymptomatic and are not known to be at increased risk for any disease. In contrast, affected individuals have varying degrees of exocrine functions alteration. CF is characterized chiefly by chronic obstruction and infection of the respiratory tract, pancreatic enzyme insufficiency, and elevated levels of sweat electrolytes. A variety of other gastrointestinal complications, as well as diabetes, can complicate the long-term management of this disorder.

Anderson first described CF as a distinct clinical entity in 1938.[5] There have been significant advances recently in identifying the genetic defect, understanding the pathophysiology involved (Mainly analysis of ion transport across the apical membrane), and therapy. This progress is best illustrated by the improved survival in CF patients. The purpose of this review is to evaluate the current knowledge of the genetic aspects, pathophysiology, the role of infection in the pathophysiology, clinical presentation, diagnostic modalities, and prophylactic and acute therapy of CF.

Cystic fibrosis is the most common lethal genetic disease in the white population.

GENETICS

The isolation of the CF transmembrane conductance regulator gene and the identification of the most common mutation, ΔF508,[4] allow comparison of the clinical cause of the disease with CF phenotype. The understanding of the basic defect in the inherited disorder, CF, required cloning of the CF gene and definition of its protein product. In the absence of direct functional information, chromosomal map positioning was used as a guide for locating the gene. Chromosomal "walking and jumping" and complementary

DNA hybridization were used to isolate DNA sequences, encompassing more than 500,000 base pairs from the CF region on the long arm of human chromosome 7. Several transcribed sequences and conserved segments were identified in this clone region, one of which corresponds to the CF gene and encompasses approximately 250,000 base pairs of genomic DNA. The putative protein coded for by cDNA for the CF locales consists of 1,480 amino acids. The three-nucleotide codon for phenylalanine located 580 amino acids from the N terminal was found to be deleted in 70% of patients with CF. The protein has been named the CF transmembrane regulator (CFTR).

This CFTR has two related motifs, each consisting of six membrane spiny regions joined by a long polypeptide chain. Two features of the cytosolic domain are important. The first is the highly charged R dominant having 60 potential sites for phosphorylation; the second is the two nucleotide binding folds that may bind or even hydrolyze ATP. The phenylalanine deletion (ΔF508) occurs in the first nucleotide binding fold.[2-4] This protein has been detected in lung, pancreas, colon, culture sweat glands, nasal polyps, placenta, liver, kidney, and parotid glands, but not in brain, adrenals, culture skin fibroblasts, or lymphoblast cell lines.[3] It has not yet been isolated, but on the basis of homology data and molecular modelling it is thought to be an ATP-dependent transport protein rather than a chloride ion channel.[4]

One of the intriguing features of the first publication on the CF gene was the apparent association between patients with pancreatic insufficiency and the ΔF508 allele. About half of the pancreatic insufficiency patients were homozygous for the deletion, whereas no pancreatic-sufficient patient had this genotype.[4] However, analysis of a German outpatient cohort did not confirm this hypothesis. Thus, there are now some doubts about whether homozygosity for ΔF508 is a useful prognosticator of a more severe course of disease.[4-7]

A key piece of evidence in the DNA clone sequence was the CF gene (ΔF508), which consisted of the finding of the same specific mutation on 70% of CF chromosomes.

One of the key pieces of evidence of the DNA clone sequence was the CF gene (ΔF508), which corresponds to the same specific mutation on 70% of CF chromosomes.[4] A recently published worldwide survey[6] of the frequency of these alleles shows considerable variation among different ethnic groups and populations. The highest frequencies are found in North European countries, with lower frequencies found in Italy, Spain, and Greece. In the United States, the frequency of this mutation is over 75%.

Early expectations that the remaining CF alleles will be limited to a small number of mutations has now faded. CF genetic analysis has shown more than 60 distinct mutations. These include missense and nonsense and RNA-splice mutations as well as deletions and insertions. Many have been found to be segregations in only one or a handful of families, whereas others are found in specific ethnic groups. It has been found that, with the exception of the predominant ΔF508 allele, CF is a genetic heterogeneous condition.

The predominant ΔF508 CF allele is easily detectable by simple electrophoresis of amplified DNA. The test can be done using blood samples, buccal cell scrapings, or chorionic villus biopsies. These molecular genetic techniques may aid in the diagnosis of questionable cases of CF, however, absence of the allele does not exclude the diagnosis.

PATHOPHYSIOLOGY

Exocrine gland dysfunction, including destruction of mucus-secreting glands with inspissated secretions and defective chloride and sodium reabsorption by serous glands, is the mechanism involved in CF. While it is clear that CF affects many organ systems, lung pathology is the most significant clinical problem, accounting for more than 95% of the mortality and the majority of morbidity from CF.[8,9]

Abnormalities in chloride (Cl^-) and sodium (Na^+) transport across the apical membrane of epithelial tissue have been identified as the most likely cellular basis of CF symptoms. The opening and closing of chloride channels in the apical membrane of epithelial cells is regulated by hormones, neurotransmitters, and enterotoxins acting through a variety of intracellular messengers, including cyclic neucleotides (AMP and GMP). The Cl^- impermeability of epithelial membrane observed in CF patients results not from a defect in the Cl^- conducting properties of the channel or in channel recruitment, but from either a defect in the key regulator of the channel, presumably phosphorous proteins, or hyperactivation of a channel-closing mechanism, presumably a protein phosphatase or a down-regulating protein kinase.[10,11] In most CF tissues examined, the β-adrenergic cAMP-mediated activation of Cl^- secretion is completed abolished.[12] In contrast, the cholinergic activation is either normal (in sweat glands) or only mildly impaired (in the airway tissue).[13] However, in the intestine Cl^- secretion is defective not only in response to cAMP but also in response to cGMP and calcium link secretagogue.[14]

While it is clear that CF affects many organ systems, lung pathology is the most significant clinical problem, accounting for more than 95% of mortality and the majority of morbidity from CF.

In most CF tissues examined, the beta-adrenergic cAMP-mediated activation of chloride secretion is completed abolished.

Sweat Glands

The human sweat gland is a tubular organ composed of two regions: the secretory coil and the reabsorptive duct. The secretory coil produces nearly isotonic sweat. How-

NaCl concentration in the sweat glands increase due to Cl$^-$ absorption blockage.

ever, as the sweat passes up to the water-impermeable duct, NaCl is absorbed and the fluid emerges hypertonic at the surface of the skin. In the coil, active Cl$^-$ transport resorbs fluid; in the duct, active Na$^+$ transport resorbs electrolytes. In each case, the counter ion appears to follow passively. Quinton and Bijman[15] found that both in vivo and in vitro CF sweat ducts have a higher transepithelial electrical potential difference than normal ducts. CF sweat ducts have a decreased Cl$^-$ permeability, and an increased transepithelial voltage results from an intact Na$^+$ absorptive mechanism in the presence of Cl$^-$ impermeability. This abnormality explains the finding that the NaCl concentration in the sweat glands increases as a result of Cl$^-$ absorption blockage. The Cl$^-$ permeability of cultured normal and CF duct cells is dependent on the presence of cholinergic (calcium-mediated) or β-adrenergic (cAMP-mediated) stimuli. In contrast, the Cl$^-$ permeability of CF ducts microperfused in vitro does not seem to be under neural or hormonal control.

Sato and Sato[16] have shown that a secretory coil of CF sweat glands also transports electrolytes abnormally. In normal sweat glands, either cholinergic or β-adrenergic agonists stimulate sweat production, although β-adrenergic-induced sweat production is one fifth the rate of cholinergic-induced sweating. Methacholine stimulates a similar rate of sweat production in both normal and CF secretory coils. In contrast, the β-adrenergic agonists, isoproterenol and theophylline, stimulate secretion in normal glands but not in CF glands. These results suggest a defect in the cAMP-mediated regulation of Cl$^-$ secretion. Thus, there is decreased Cl$^-$ transport in the duct and secretory coil with inhibition of fluid absorption, resulting in an increase in NaCl in sweat.

Airway Tissue

Transepithelial electrolyte transport controls the quality and composition of respiratory tract fluids, thus it is important in effecting normal mucociliary clearance.[13] The clinical observation that CF airway secretions are thick and dehydrated led Knowles et al.[11] to study the electrolyte transport by CF respiratory epithelium. They found that in vivo voltage across the upper (nasal) and lower (tracheal and bronchial) airway epithelium is higher in CF patients. This study, with the subsequent observation that transepithelial Cl$^-$ fluxes are decreased in excised nasal polyps, indicates that CF airway epithelium is relatively impermeable to Cl$^-$ along the apical membrane.

The increased epithelial voltage in CF airway epithelium

and the dehydration of airway secretions raise the possibility that Na^+ absorption may also be abnormal in CF, but this has not been completely elucidated.[17]

LUNG DISEASE

The precise evolution of lung disease in CF remains undefined. Evidence suggests that infection is a secondary, but significant, process in the pathogenesis. The early changes in CF are inflammatory and noninfective. The morphologic changes of dilatation and hypertrophy of the bronchial glands are followed by mucous plugging. Infection soon follows and contributes to ongoing tissue damage, manifested by bronchiectasis, peribronchial fibrosis, and airflow obstruction. The primary pathogens in CF are *Pseudomonas aeruginosa* and *Staphylococcus aureus*. *Haemophilus influenzae* has been cultured in 10–30% of patients, usually in those with more than 10 years of the disease. Other potential pathogens occasionally isolated include *Escherichia coli*, *Klebsiella pneumoniae*, and *Mycoplasma pneumoniae*.[18,19]

It is unclear how mucosal ion transport abnormalities are related to the role of bacteria in CF. It has frequently been suggested that impaired mucosal clearance and Cl^- transfer dysfunction may be the crucial mechanisms in bacterial colonization. Intact mucosal defenses and the combination of mechanical clearance, biochemical environment, and local immunity would normally prevent bacterial binding and subsequent colonization; some mechanical–chemical infection-induced injury would have to occur before bacteria would adhere.[20]

Ciliary dysfunction, as well as alteration of the viscoelastic properties of the tracheobronchial secretions, are the prominent features of CF. In addition, there is evidence that some of the immunologic abnormalities found in patients with CF are part of a hyperimmune process, whereas others, such as alteration of immunoglobulins and complement, decreased pulmonary macrophage activity, and lymphocyte hyperresponsiveness, represent an acquired impairment of immune function. Certain impairments are most likely due to toxic and proteolytic damage inflicted by proteolytic enzymes from stimulated neutrophils and by bacterial toxins and elastase.[21]

Mucosal injuries will inhibit mucocilary clearance and structural airway wall defects will impair the effectiveness of cough in eliminating bacterial and proteolytic material, whereas a spectrum of bacterial and host-derived factors will impair immunologic defenses. Once this vicious cycle is established, the chronicity of the bacterial infection may progressively relate to a continuous increase in nonspecific

The primary pathogens in CF are **Pseudomonas aeruginosa** *and* **Staphylococcus aureus.**

Respiratory viral infections damage respiratory mucosa, facilitating adherence and colonization by PA.

damage and ultimately may become independent of the basic, inherent mucosal ion transport defect. Although this basic and CF-specific defect should be seen as the initiator of the disease process, it may then progressively lose its importance in perpetrating later disease stages.[22]

A considerable variability in the time of onset and severity of active infection exists among patients. Although this variability can be attributed to some inpatient differences in the expression of the basic mucosal defect, it may also be caused by the chance occurrence of additional exogenous injuries in combination with inherent defects by initial bacterial colonization. Several triggering factors have been postulated. Respiratory viral infection has been documented to produce damage to respiratory mucosa by facilitating adherence and colonization by *P. aeruginosa*. For example, in infants with CF, respiratory syncitial viral infection can initiate early, severe, and persistent respiratory disease. Such viral infections probably promote bacterial colonization.[23] Later on, this will help to establish lung damage. Other microorganisms may contribute directly to lung injury; for example, *S. aureus* is frequently responsible for the first episode of bronchial pulmonary bacterial infection in CF, which is then followed by *P. aeruginosa* colonization. This transition from initial staphylococcal to subsequent and chronic *P. aeruginosa* infection is at least in part based on the affinity of *P. aeruginosa* for damage epithelial surfaces, but may also be facilitated by selective initial antibiotic intervention. The mechanism by which *S. aureus* or other microorganisms can set the stage for colonization with *P. aeruginosa* are not clear, but injury to the respiratory mucosa may have a crucial role in this characteristic sequence of bacterial lung disease.[21,23]

The sputums of patients with CF colonized exclusively with *S. aureus* contains elevated concentrations of free elastase, which has proteolytic activity on fibronectin. Loss of cell surface fibronectin has been shown to result in increased adherence of *P. aeruginosa* to epithelial cells.[24] Thus, a sequential alteration of mucosal surface by elastase may play a role in the characteristic sequence of bacterial colonization: first, *S. aureus* binding and inflicting damage to cell surface, then *P. aeruginosa* adhering to the surface deprived of fibronectin.

Poor nutritional status, frequent in CF, is also a factor in enhancing bacterial binding to the respiratory epithelium.[25] Other factors that produce mucosal damage include exposure to tobacco smoke (passive smoking) and air pollution, which promote bacterial colonization in CF but have not been investigated.

Bacterial Colonization

Bacterial colonization is characterized by the expression of a mucoid phenotype of *P. aeruginosa* that produces copious quantities of alginate, an extracellular polysaccharide. It is still unclear whether initial colonization occurs by a mucoid strain or whether a nonmucoid to mucoid transformation occurs subsequently in the lower respiratory tract of the host.[26] Alginate production is almost exclusively found in *P. aeruginosa* strains isolated from patients with CF. Alginate forms a large-volume matrix around the microorganism, thereby producing a alginate-protective microcolony of bacteria. The sheer volume of such a microcolony prevents pulmonary macrophages and neutrophils from ingesting the bacteria and also impairs opsonization. This alginate not only protects *P. aeruginosa* against phagocytosis, but also reduces the mechanical efficacy of the mucociliary and cough mechanisms. The large hydrated volumes of the matrix itself may reduce the effectiveness of the ciliary beating and obstruct small airways. Furthermore, arginase interacts with mucin glycoproteins in the presence of calcium ions, thereby leading to an increase in the viscosity of the bronchopulmonary secretions. Thus, expression of the mucoid phenotype of *P. aeruginosa* most likely carries the major responsibility for the chronic measure of the infection. Although it has no direct toxic effect alginate may contribute to tissue damage by localizing bacterial toxins, thereby concentrating injury in discrete regions.[17-21,23-26]

P. aeruginosa secretes factors that contribute to tissue damage and, by impairing several aspects of host immunity, are responsible for the chronic nature of the infection. Secreted elastase and alkaline proteases degrade tissue proteins such as elastin collagen and basement membrane laminin. Also, cilia inhibitory factors, namely PYo compounds and phenazine derivatives, impair mucociliary transport by allowing increased mucin release from respiratory epithelium, thus inhibiting ciliary motility. *P. aeruginosa* also has a profound effect on the immunologic defenses of the host. Secreted proteases cleave immunoglobulins and inhibit the antibacterial action in neutrophils, and exotoxin A is toxic to pulmonary macrophages.[27] Finally, *P. aeruginosa* undergoes an environmental adaptation to CF lung characterized by changes in somatic antigens and serum sensitivity. Such changes will have implications for disease progression and antibiotic susceptibility, and are responsible for the emergence of multiresistant strains.

In an attempt to explain various immunologic findings of the host response, several investigators have proposed

It is unclear whether initial colonization occurs by mucoid strain or whether nonmucoid-to-mucoid transformation occurs subsequently in the lower respiratory tract.

a hypothesis of the type III hypersensitive reaction in order to make a correlation between the *P. aeruginosa* infection and the lung damage (Fig. 1).[8]

P. aeruginosa may supply the antigens for an immune complex disease, which by means of complement activation and generation of chemotactic split products ultimately causes a release of lysosomal enzymes and oxygen radicals that stimulate neutrophils.[22] Extravascular formation of immune complex disease has been documented in the respiratory tract of CF patients. It has been suggested that this immune complex is produced in the lung of infected patients. Longitudinal variations of immune complex activity in sputum and serum correlate with alterations in lung function during the clinical course of the disease.[28] Furthermore, high antibody levels against *P. aeruginosa* exoproducts indicate a pure clinical state and severe lung function impairment. The key event in the immune complex formation–tissue damage sequence is the release of lysosomal enzymes from stimulated neutrophils. This host-derived proteolytic activity may be responsible both for the tissue damage and for facilitating the persistence of infection.

In summary, the mechanisms described will result in sig-

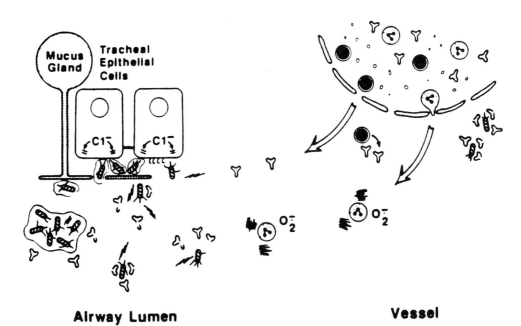

Airway Lumen   **Vessel**

FIG. 1   Theory of the relationship of respiratory *P. aeruginosa* infections and defective chloride transport of epithelial cells. An abnormal glycoprotein encases *P. aeruginosa*, preventing opsophagocytic clearance. *P. aeruginosa* elastase cleaves immunoglobulins and inhibits neutrophil-derived elastase, and toxic oxygen products (e.g., O_2^-) contribute to the destructive lesion of the airways. From Fick RB Jr: Pathogenesis of the *Pseudomonas* lung lesion in cystic fibrosis. Chest 96:159, 1989. With permission.

nificant structural, ultrastructural, and immunologic injury.

The chronic presence of bacteria stimulates and attracts polymorphonuclear neutrophils of the lung. These polymorphonuclear neutrophils produce chemotactic split products. In advanced disease stages, more than 99% of the cells from bronchoalveolar lavage of CF lungs are neutrophils. Release of oxygen radicals by lysosomal enzymes from the neutrophils is maximally stimulated by "frustrated phagocytosis," so named because of inability of the neutrophils to engulf the large, alginate-protected microcolonies of P. aeruginosa.[29] The insufficient neutralization of neutrophil-derived elastase and other proteases normally inactivated by the system of plasma-base and bronchial inhibitors is probably responsible for the progression of the lung disease and the ongoing tissue damage in CF subjects.

The elastolytic activity of the sputum of CF patients is significantly higher than that of the sputum of patients with chronic bronchitis and uninfected controls. This high enzymatic activity correlates with the advanced disease stage. Any long-term exposure of lung tissue to proteolytic enzyme will ultimately result in degradation of connective tissue. This ongoing proteolytic damage to the bronchial tissue results in progressive destruction of airway wall structures. In fact, bronchiectasis remains the predominant finding in the studies of lung pathology. Lungs in advanced disease stages reveal gross alterations in anatomic lung volume proportions, mainly a marked increase in airway volume proportionate to the volume of parenchyma. While the proportion of bronchial volume remains around 4% of the lobar volume in healthy lungs, it is increased 10–20% in CF. Occasionally, bronchiectatic airways can occupy 50% of the entire lung volume.[30] This anatomic volume disproportion varies significantly between the upper and the lower lobes. In particular, the increased proportion of bronchial volume together with a corresponding reduction in lung parenchyma is more marked in the upper lobes than in the lower ones; furthermore, cystic lesions occur predominantly in upper lung regions.

In most cases, bronchiectasis is present beyond the first year of life and increases with disease progression and age. In contrast, obstructive inflammatory mucosal edema and accumulation of mucopurulent secretions are equally common in all age groups beyond the neonate. Other obstructive lesions, such as stenosis of small airways due to fibrosis and chronic inflammatory changes, are predominantly found in older patients.[31] The significance and prevalence of bronchial gland enlargement remains controversial. Finally, lung pathology beyond the neonatal period has the

In advanced disease stages, more than 99% of the cells from bronchoalveolar lavage of CF lungs are neutrophils.

In most cases, bronchiectasis is present beyond the first year of life and increases with disease progression and age.

following characteristics:

1. Chronic bronchitis, bronchiolitis, and mucopurulent airway plugging which are found in all age groups.

2. Bronchiectatic dilatation of the airways at the expense of lung parenchyma, a dominating component of lung pathology, which increases gradually with age or with progression of disease.

3. Bronchial stenosis, scarring, pneumonia, and nonobligatory changes, which are found mostly in advanced disease stages.

IMPAIRED PULMONARY FUNCTION

The destructive changes in lung parenchyma reflect changes in the pulmonary function, as the pattern of lung function abnormalities in patients with CF is essentially one of progressive intrathoracic airway obstruction.[32] A variable component of bronchospasm frequently contributes to these abnormalities. Obstructive lesions begin and persist in the small, peripheral airways, leading to increased airflow resistance, hyperinflation, entrapment of gas, uneven distribution of ventilation, and owing to ventilation/perfusion inequalities impairment of gas exchange.[33]

The most significant anatomic feature, bronchiectatic airway dilatation, does not correlate with the physiologic picture of the disease (Fig. 2). The maximum expiratory flow volume occurs in CF patients having an abnormally large supramaximal expiratory flow volume transiently. Early expired flow from the central intrathoracic airways directly relates to the emptying of the ectatic bronchi that were dilated by the preceding inspiration. This transience illustrates one of the two mechanical consequences of airway wall instability, namely increased airway distensibility. Unstable airways, distended by the negative intrathoracic pressure of an inspiration, will collapse when subjected to the positive pressure of a forced expiration. Such collapse is evident from the isovolume pressure flow curve, which demonstrates a negative effort dependency and bending of the ascending part of the normally low alveolar pressures. From a physiologic viewpoint, lung disease in CF can be understood as a variable combination of peripheral, partially bronchospastic, airway obstruction and central, mainly bronchiectatic, airway wall instability. The unstable central airways are distended by a deep inspiration; as abnormally compliant structures, they then contribute mark-

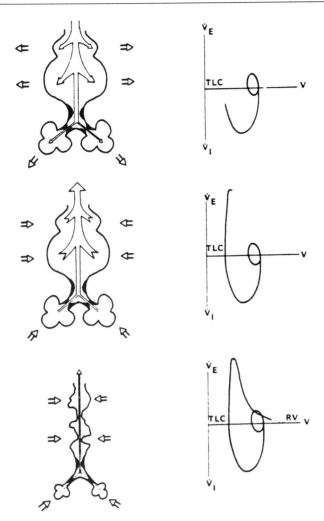

FIG. 2   Airway instability concept. (Left) Lung disease in CF as a combination of central instability and peripheral obstruction. (Right) Corresponding flow–volume tracings. (Top) Inspiration. (Middle) Early forced expiration. (Bottom) Late forced expiration. V, volume; V_1, inspiratory flow; $\dot{V}_E$, expiratory flow; TLC, total lung capacity; RV, residual volume. From Zach MS: Lung disease in cystic fibrosis—an updated concept. Pediatr Pulmonol 8:188, 1990. With permission.

edly to increased early expired volumes and flow rates. Thereafter, they are compressed by the positive transthoracic pressure, adding a dynamic component to the possible causes of airway obstruction in CF. This airway instability concept offers an explanation for the typical shape of the maximum expiratory flow–volume curve in advanced disease stages, where a high peak flow rate contrasts with a severely compromised end expiratory flow rate.[33,34]

Bronchial wall stability depends on intact wall structures, but is also maintained and regulated by bronchial smooth muscle tone. Increased bronchial smooth muscle tone may therefore contribute to airway obstruction and can also partially compensate for the mechanical consequences of airway wall destruction. This mechanism offers an explanation for paradoxical improvement of lung function after bronchial provocation testing in patients with CF.[35]

No systematic studies have correlated airway wall instability with age or disease stage. Since airway instability is the consequence of bronchiectatic airway wall destruction, one can assume that it will increase with age and certainly with disease progression, although this pathologic process may be superimposed onto the natural age-related cause of the disease.

In summary, bronchiectatic airway wall instability in CF patients may have implications for the clinical course of the disease, interpretation of lung function tests, and the respiratory effects of regional management. In addition, it may be the determining factor in the effectiveness of bronchodilator medication and in the efficacy of coughing and forced expirations in clearing intrabronchial secretions.[22]

OTHER ORGAN INVOLVEMENT

The gastrointestinal tract, mainly exocrine glands of the pancreas and the hepatobiliary tree, is affected in CF patients.

The gastrointestinal tract, mainly the exocrine glands of the pancreas, liver, and hepatobiliary tree, is also affected in CF patients. The secretory defect of epithelial tissue that causes viscid secretions probably accounts for most pathologic lesions. In addition, abnormal electrolyte transport affects the gastrointestinal tract in a variety of ways. In the small intestines and colon, defective Cl^- transport appears to lead to relative dehydration on the luminal surface, producing viscid intestinal mucus and a high protein concentration of CF meconium. Similarly, hepatobiliary secretions contain the highest concentration of bile salts, despite reduced total bile salt secretions.

Characteristic morphologic features of the CF pancreas include marked acinar atrophy, fibrosis, and fatty replacement. There is often inspissation of secretions in ducts and acini. Accumulation of secretory material within the duct is an early characteristic of CF. Obstruction that causes intraductal dilatation, progressive degradation, and atrophy of the acini follows. Pancreatic cyst formation and ductal calcification may be due to a similar pathologic process. A false impairment of pancreatic fluid secretion appears to be the primary phenomenon in CF. It has also been shown that pancreatic secretions in CF patients contain significantly higher concentrations of protein in comparison to pancreatic secretions of matched controls. Since total protein output is not increased, hyperconcentration of protein appears to be a direct result of a primary defect of fluid secretion. Protein hyperconcentration appears to predispose CF patients to protein precipitation and obstruction within a small pancreatic duct, which in turn produces pancreatic acinar atrophy and fibrosis.

Other organs that are affected are the liver and the hepatobiliary tree. The incidence of pathology increases with age, and in adults may grow to 30% or more. Improved Cl^- secretion disturbs bile production, resulting in decreased volume. Bile plugs commonly found in the portal tract probably represent an essential abnormality of the liver in CF. Focal biliary fibrosis has also been described. Obstruction or stenosis of the extrahepatic bile ducts and fatty infiltration from hepatocytes can lead to portal hypertension and varices. Obstruction of the biliary system may be seen in the extrahepatic ducts and much later in the intrahepatic ductal system.[36]

CLINICAL PRESENTATION

Clinically, CF is characterized by chronic pulmonary disease, pancreatic insufficiency, and elevated sweat electrolytes. CF is the most frequent cause of chronic lung disease and progressive pulmonary failure associated with other organ disease (e.g., pancreatic insufficiency) in childhood. Table 1 summarizes the clinical manifestations of CF. Most cases are diagnosed in childhood. Because affected individuals now routinely live beyond their 20th birthday, CF is encountered more often by physicians dealing with adults.[37] While some of the symptoms, such as increased shortness of breath and hemoptysis, will develop in line with progressing lung damage, others, such as cough and sputum production, may be a presenting feature. Lung damage is not, therefore, a prerequisite for respiratory symptoms, and it may well be that the basic defect and its physiologic consequences are as important as the structural changes. Airway secretions are very difficult to collect and analyze in symptomatic patients, so the effect of these changes is unknown. As the disease progresses, bacterial colonization develops, followed by an inflammatory response that itself produces further changes in airway secretions. The net effect is that both the volume and viscosity of secretions is increased and mucociliary clearance is impaired.

Coughing is predominantly initiated by rapidly adapting

Because affected individuals now may live beyond their 20th birthday, CF is encountered more often by physicians who treat adults.

TABLE 1 Clinical
Manifestations
of Cystic
Fibrosis

Secretory defect

High sweat chloride
concentrations
   Hyponatremia
   Hypochloremia
   Metabolic alkalosis
Abnormally viscous
secretions
   Lungs
      Recurrent pneumonia
      Chronic lung disease
   Pancreas
      Exocrine pancreatic
         insufficiency
      Pancreatitis
      Glucose intolerance
      Adult onset diabetes
         mellitus
   Intestine
      Meconium ileus
      Distal intestinal
         obstruction
   Hepatobiliary
      Focal biliary fibrosis
      Multilobular cirrhosis
      Cholelithiasis
   Vas deferens
      Male infertility

irritant receptors in the trachea and large bronchi. The combination of persistent infection and mucosal damage can lead to local inflammation and increased mucosecretion, which itself can lead to coughing. It is interesting that inhaled electrolyte solutions are powerful cough stimulants and that the lower the Cl^- ion concentration, the more coughing is provoked. Conversely, an increase in the Cl^- concentration of the inhaled solutions reduces the cough frequency. Furthermore, the cough receptors appear to be sensitive to local electrical changes. Changes in Cl^- permeability and surface changes in the airway may therefore be important variables in the production of coughing in CF.

Another symptom is the presence of wheezing or airway airflow obstruction, which is caused by a combination of intraluminal secretions, mucosal edema, airway smooth muscle contraction, small airway obliteration, and major airway distortion. While some of these abnormalities, such as the obliteration and distortion, are the end result of widespread irreversible lung damage, other factors are produced by inflammation and are therefore potentially reversible. The inflammation is largely due to infection, and the release of chemotactic inflammatory mediators will affect the mucous secretion and vascular permeability of smooth muscle tone. Increased airway reactivity as the result of an allergic IgE-mediated inflammatory reaction may be a prominent symptom. Allergy to *Aspergillus fumigatus* is a particular problem, causing increased frequency in mucous plugging and eosinophilic infiltration in CF.

CF patients may also show minor blood streaking in the sputum, although major hemoptysis is unusual and is largely restricted to patients with severe lung damage. Occasional coexisting liver disease with blood clotting disorders or hypersplenism with a reduced number of platelets may play an important role. There is an increased risk of pneumothorax as the lung damage increases and greater changes in the pleural pressure are required for normal breathing. In addition, there are local areas of pulmonary damage and cystic changes. These complications tend to occur in young adults, and they may also be related to poor nutritional and weakening of the connective tissue.

Breathlessness is an important subjective symptom, and may be due to a combination of processes involving airflow, gas exchange, respiratory muscles, and hemodynamics. Repeated infection causes inflammatory obstruction in small airways with areas of atelectasis intermingled with areas of overt distension, together with widespread bronchiectasis, scar emphysema, and localized fibrosis. These structural changes affect the regional distribution of ventilation and perfusion with resultant hypoxemia. Hemodynamic abnormalities develop first only upon exercise, subsequently on minimal exertion, and then at rest. Cor pulmonale develops in the preterminal stages. Only in severe disease (i.e., an FEV_1 [forced expiratory volume after 1 second] of less than 50% of predicted, or a DL_{CO} [diffusin capacity for carbon monoxide] of less than 65%) is exercise performance impaired.

Respiratory muscle function is impaired by changes in chest wall configuration as the residual volume increases; this is aggravated by the increase in respiratory work due to a combination of airflow obstruction, reduced compliance, and an increased minute ventilation. Hypoxia and malnutrition also impaired muscle function.

Sleep is associated with a significant degree of nocturnal oxygen desaturation in CF patients, particularly during REM sleep. In general, the degree of desaturation is related to the severity of the underlying lung disease.[38] Hypopnea is observed with no evidence of significant apnea or snoring, however, the mechanism of desaturation is thought to be due to changes in the distribution of ventilation and perfusion with episodes of superimposed hypoventilation.

Sleep, particularly REM sleep, is associated with a significant degree of nocturnal oxygen desaturation in CF patients.

GASTROINTESTINAL MANIFESTATIONS

About 85% of CF patients have severe loss of pancreatic acinar tissue that results in inadequate secretion of digestive enzymes and malabsorption. These individuals present with large, bulky, greasy stools and poor weight gain or frank weight loss. They may develop manifestations of fat-soluble vitamin deficiencies. About 15–20% of CF patients retain functional acinar tissue sufficient to digest and absorb nutrients normally and do not require pancreatic enzyme supplementation. They have a far better overall prognosis than patients with pancreatic insufficiency and usually do not develop some of the other gastrointestinal complications such as hepatobiliary disease and distal intestinal obstruction syndrome.[39] Among patients with pancreatic insufficiency, recurrent pancreatitis may be a problem mainly because of ductal obstruction and acinar release of enzymes. Progressive pancreatic fibrosis ultimately disrupts isolated pancreatic cell function. At least 30% of patients with pancreatic insufficiency have an abnormal tolerance to glucose loads. Frank diabetes is less frequent and tends to be correlated with the course of the disease.[40]

The major intestinal manifestations are the result of partial or complete obstruction of the intestinal lumen. Ob-

At least 30% of patients with pancreatic insufficiency have an abnormal tolerance to glucose loads.

struction may occur in utero or at any time during the patient's life. Intestinal presentation of CF includes meconium ileus, meconium peritonitis, intestinal atresia, unexplained intestinal obstruction, and rectal prolapse.

Hepatic abnormalities include gallbladder involvement (in 45% of patients) and fatty liver (in 15–40% of patients), as well as other complications of focal biliary fibrosis and multilobular cirrhosis. Intrahepatic and extrahepatic biliary calculi are a major complication in CF patients. Cirrhosis is the second most severe and clinically important problem in CF. It may be the first manifestation of liver disease and be present despite only mild abnormality of liver enzymes. Although cirrhosis rarely causes hepatocellular failure, it is associated with portal hypertension and esophageal varices in 2–5% of patients.

NUTRITIONAL MANIFESTATIONS

Patients with CF are at risk for nutritional deficiencies by three main mechanisms: malabsorption, increased requirements to compensate for the effects of chronic lung disease and perhaps also to meet the needs arising from the basic metabolic disease in CF, and decreased food intake resulting from illness. All three factors contribute to the frequent development of severe malnutrition. The fact that energy and nutrient intake is insufficient to meet requirements accounts for poor weight gain and growth, delayed puberty, muscle wasting, and vitamin, mineral, essentially fatty acid, and taurine deficiencies.[40] On theoretic grounds, improved nutrition should enhance respiratory muscle strength and immunity, and may therefore have important long-term effects on the state of the lungs and ultimately on prognosis. Retrospectively, a cross-section of studies have already documented a correlation between good nutrition and improvement in both lung function and survival.[40]

DIAGNOSIS

The diagnosis of CF is made by a combination of clinical features and sweat Cl^- determinations. Clinical features include pulmonary manifestations, gastrointestinal manifestations, and/or a history of CF in the immediate family. In addition, the sweat Cl^- level should be greater than 60 mEq/L.[41] It is recommended that sweat Cl^- determinations be done according to the method of Gibson and Cooke.[42] Pilocarpine is introduced into the skin by iontophoresis to produce localized sweating. The perspiration is collected for 30 minutes and then analyzed. Because proper analysis requires meticulous adherence to protocol, laboratories routinely accustomed to performing the analysis should be used. This may avoid inaccurate sweat Cl⁻ determinations and diagnoses either falsely positive or negative.

Sweat Cl⁻ determinations should be interpreted together with the clinical scenario. A small percentage of patients have clinical features suggestive of CF but normal sweat Cl⁻ levels. Suggested criteria for the diagnosis of CF in this subgroup of patients are presented in Table 2.[43] A subset of the normal population may have sweat Cl⁻ levels greater than 60 mEq/L. Various clinical conditions may alter sweat Cl⁻, including untreated adrenal insufficiency, renal diabetes insipidus, fucosidosis, and untreated hypothyroidism, all of which are associated with elevated levels. Drug therapy with steroids, β-agonists, and theophylline may lower sweat Cl⁻ determinations.[44] Therefore, factors in addition to sweat Cl⁻ must be considered for the diagnosis of CF.

Advances in technology have provided alternative methods for the diagnosis of CF. Measurement of the bioelectric potential difference across respiratory epithelia reveals the

---

TABLE 2   Diagnostic Criteria for Cystic Fibrosis

Major criteria
  Sweat chloride concentration above 60 mmol/L before age 20 years or above 80 mmol/L in an adult.
  Chronic obstructive pulmonary disease with pseudomonas airway infection.
  Unexplained obstructive azoospermia.
Minor criteria
  Sweat chloride concentration above 40 mmol/L before age 20 years or above 60 mmol/L in an adult.
  Family history of classic cystic fibrosis.
  Exocrine pancreatic insufficiency before age 20 years.
  Unexplained chronic obstructive pulmonary disease before age 20 years.
  Unexplained azoospermia (demonstrated by semen analysis without scrotal examination).
Minor criteria candidates
  Unexplained recurrent pancreatitis in adolescent or young adult.
  Unexplained biliary cirrhosis in child, adolescent, or young adult.
  Unexplained cholelithiasis in adolescent or young adult.
Diagnosis is established by the presence of two minor findings or by one major finding and one minor finding. The two criteria used for diagnosis must involve different organ systems.

From Stern RC, Boat TF, Doershuk CF: Obstructive azoospermia as a diagnostic criterion for the cystic fibrosis syndrome. Lancet 1:1401, 1982. © The Lancet Ltd. With permission.

---

difference to be increased in patients with CF.[45] DNA analysis to detect the CF gene may be pursued in questionable cases.[46] Antenatal diagnosis by analysis of amniotic fluid and DNA probes may be pursued in families with a history of CF.[47] Neonatal screening may identify patients with CF, however, it is not recommended on a routine basis.[48]

TREATMENT

The primary manifestation of CF in adults is that of pulmonary disease. Thus, we will concentrate on therapeutic options for treatment of pulmonary involvement in this chronic, progressive disease.

Antibiotics

In addition to the controversy over length and timing of therapy, the route of antibiotic administration remains in question.

The introduction of penicillin to therapy of CF patients more than 40 years ago markedly improved the prognosis of those patients who are plagued initially with *S. aureus* infection and colonization of the airways and later in the disease course by *P. aeruginosa*.[49] Controversy remains over prophylaxis to prevent colonization versus therapy only for acute deterioration in respiratory status. In addition to the controversy over length and timing of therapy, the route of antibiotic administration remains in question. It is difficult to attribute all improvement to antibiotic therapy alone, as hospitalization may provide more intensive therapy, including chest physiotherapy, bronchodilators, improved nutrition, and compliance with therapy.

There are no firm data to mandate *Staphylococcus* prophylaxis.[50,51] Although staphylococcal infection is thought to be part of the inciting event for lung destruction. There are those who propose eradication of *Staphylococcus* when it is initially isolated from the sputum, in addition to antistaphylococcal coverage in later stages of the disease usually treated with antipseudomonal therapy alone.[51] One of the few placebo-controlled trials examining antistaphylococcal prophylaxis included only 17 patients, 10 of whom were colonized with *S. aureus*, 13 with *H. influenzae*, and 11 with *P. aeruginosa*.[52] They found that oral cephalexin decreased the frequency of respiratory illness and colonization with *S. aureus* and *H. influenzae*, with the majority demonstrating improvement in spirometric testing and weight gain. However, patients initially colonized with *Pseudomonas* tended to have an increase in mucoid strains and disease severity; due to the small number of patients it is difficult to attribute deterioration to therapy in these patients. Currently the Cystic Fibrosis Foundation is performing a placebo-controlled trial to determine the efficacy of long-term anti-staphylococcal prophylaxis in CF patients.

Despite the lack of well-controlled placebo trials, the current standard of care includes antipseudomonal therapy during acute exacerbations. *P. aeruginosa* colonizes 80% of patients with CF.[53] Antibiotic therapy has improved the 10-year survival rate in CF patients colonized with *Pseudomonas* to 90% compared to a previous 54% 5-year survival.[54] Intravenous antipseudomonal therapy has demonstrated a decrease in sputum organism colony count[55,56] and clinical improvement not necessarily related to sputum volume or organism colony count.[56] However, the decrease in *Pseudomonas* colony count with therapy is transient despite continued improvement in pulmonary function testing,[57] and therefore may not be a good indicator of response to therapy. Oral antipseudomonal agents have been used to treat acute deterioration in pulmonary status in CF and have demonstrated to be perhaps even more effective than intravenous antibiotics in improvement of pulmonary function at 4 to 6 weeks without increase of resistant organisms at this time.[58]

The question of "maintenance" or prophylactic therapy is not answered. Szaff and colleagues[59] observed outcome of CF patients colonized with *P. aeruginosa* over a 4-year period. Those treated with periodic prophylactic therapy (β-lactam/tobramycin or tobramycin alone) had an increase in survival compared to patients treated for acute deterioration only (82% versus 54%) as well as improved pulmonary function. Colonization did not necessarily reflect lack of response to therapy as 33% remained colonized with *P. aeruginosa*. The administration of intravenous antibiotics may be accomplished through hospital admission or home care without significant increase in morbidity related to intravenous catheters. Factors that may alter this decision include patient support and the availability of close medical follow-up. The development of oral antipseudomonal agents may alter future prophylactic therapy, although there is concern over development of resistance with long-term use.[60]

Regardless of home or hospital administration of intravenous antibiotics, the expense of intravenous therapy in the context of this chronic disease had led to the search for a more economical, less invasive manner of antibiotic administration. Inhaled antibiotic therapy has been explored as a therapeutic option. Advantages to this route of administration in the case of aminoglycosides include higher sputum concentration compared to intravenous delivery of the medication and less systemic toxicity. However, delivery of the medication to the airway may be impeded by secre-

The current standard of care includes antipseudomonas therapy during acute exacerbations.

*Colonization does not necessarily reflect lack of response to therapy, as 33% of patients in one study remained colonized with **Pseudomonas aeruginosa**.*

tions, airway resistance, and the mode of delivery, which affects particle size (i.e., particles smaller than 2 μm are delivered to alveoli).[61]

Studies have addressed therapy of acute respiratory deterioration in CF with aerosolized antibiotics. Schaad and colleagues[62] randomized 87 patients with CF to intravenous ceftazadime and amikacin versus the same regimen plus aerosolized amikacin during an exacerbation of their pulmonary disease. Serum levels were adequate in both groups, with an increased sputum concentration of amikacin in the group receiving nebulized medication (10.3 μg/ml) compared to those receiving intravenous therapy alone (1.7 μg/ml). The colonization rate with *P. aeruginosa* was initially decreased in the group receiving inhaled amikacin (70% to 41%); however, 4 to 6 weeks later, colonization was back to baseline and there was no difference in clinical outcome of the two groups at that time. Similarly, a short-term placebo cross-over trial with inhaled tobramycin in older patients did not demonstrate a benefit in pulmonary function, bacterial density, or clinical outcome.[63] Cooper and colleagues[64] looked at the benefit of high-dose intravenous therapy (ticarcillin/tobramycin) versus high-dose inhaled therapy (carbenicillin/tobramycin) in 18 patients with acute respiratory exacerbations. They found similar clinical improvement in both treatment groups acutely. This raises the issue of the necessity of hospitalization during deterioration in pulmonary status.

Prophylactic inhaled antibiotic therapy has also been a subject of investigation. The addition of inhaled antistaphylococcal therapy to oral therapy has demonstrated no clear-cut benefit over oral antistaphylococcal therapy alone with similar patient clinical status and colonization.[65] Prophylaxis with inhaled antipseudomonal therapy in the form of monotherapy or combination therapy such as carbenicillin and gentamicin resulted in stability or improvement of pulmonary function testing in patients with CF compared to control patients.[66,67] However, as with intravenous therapy the problem of drug-resistant organisms developed (33%).[67] Again, further studies should be pursued to determine long-term benefit to the patient.

With development of antipseudomonal therapy, there is increasing concern for the development of resistant organisms in the debilitated patient with CF. Drug therapy may promote change in colony properties of *P. aeruginosa* from nonmucoid to mucoid. Additionally, analysis of CF patients in Toronto during the years of 1970 to 1981 demonstrated that *P. aeruginosa* colonization remained stable at 70–80% with an increase of the multiply drug-resistant *P. cepacia* from 10 to 18%. Those patients colonized with *P.*

cepacia had an increased mortality rate compared to those patients without this colonization.[22]

There are a few caveats concerning antibiotic therapy in patients with CF. These patients may require higher doses of antibiotics compared to other patients due to a variety of factors, including differing pharmacokinetics, lower sputum drug concentrations and activity due to purulence and pH of the sputum, and change in organism sensitivity with therapy. It is recommended that serum levels of aminoglycosides in particular be followed in order to maintain therapeutic concentrations. Piperacillin has been associated with a serum sickness-like syndrome in 24–72% of patients with CF; therefore the use of this drug might be reconsidered. The addition of clavulinic acid to ticarcillin may not offer an advantage in patients with CF as the concentration is not enough to restore the activity of ticarcillin to normal and it may also induce chromosomal β-lactamase; therefore ticarcillin alone may suffice.[68] Imipenem[68] and aztreonam[69] have been shown to be acceptable antipseudomonal agents in CF.

In summary, there should be a scientific basis for antibiotic therapy rather than empiric therapy during pulmonary decompensation in CF due to the potentially lethal consequence of infection with resistant organisms such as *P. cepacia*.[50] Other organisms that may have to be dealt with in increasing frequency include rapidly growing mycobacteria, *Mycoplasma pneumonia*, respiratory synestial virus, and fungal infection. It is recommended that antibiotics to treat acute pulmonary deterioration in CF be chosen based on sputum culture results. The question of antibiotic prophylaxis is unclear.

Cystic fibrosis patients may require higher doses of antibiotics compared to other patients due to a variety of factors, including differing pharmacokinetics, lower sputum drug concentrations and activity due to purulence and pH of the sputum, and change in organism sensitivity with therapy.

Bronchodilators

Bronchodilator therapy along with antibiotics and aggressive pulmonary toilet remain standard therapy during deterioration of respiratory status in CF. Hordvik and colleagues[70] in following patients at close intervals as outpatients or during hospitalization for pulmonary exacerbations determined that the response to bronchodilator therapy varies according to the status of the disease process and that objective evidence of improvement on spirometric testing may be lacking during acute deterioration. This, however, should not discourage use of bronchodilators. Besides the beneficial effect of decreasing airway hyperreactivity the potential benefits of increasing ciliary motility and clearing secretions should be considered. Similar to patients with chronic bronchitis, it has been demonstrated

Besides beneficial effects of decreasing airway hyperreactivity, potential benefits of bronchodilators include increasing ciliary motility and aid in clearance of secretions should be considered.

that bronchodilator therapy increases ciliary motility in patients with CF.[71]

Potential negative effects of bronchodilators in CF have also been studied. Bronchodilators may reduce efficacy of cough by stabilizing bronchomotor tone and decreasing the ability of airways to withstand the dynamic compression during forced expiration, thus increasing large airway collapse.[72] It is recommended that the change in end-expiratory flow be monitored to avoid inhibition of effective cough.

SECRETION CLEARANCE

The proposed benefit of chest physiotherapy (CPT) is to clear secretions and thus decrease airway obstruction and proteolytic tissue damage by the secretions. CPT, however, requires the commitment of time and effort of family. Although CPT is standard in the care in CF, the question of this commitment versus patient benefits was explored by De Boeck and colleagues.[73] The acute benefit of CPT was compared to cough alone with no significant functional response and no correlation with volume of sputum production found. However, others have shown increased sputum clearance with CPT compared to cough alone.[74] Other techniques of clearing secretions include the forced expiration technique (expiration from lower lung volumes) and autogenic drainage, both of which require training and coordination to perform, as well as intraluminal positive expiratory pressure, which acts to open airways to improve clearance of secretions.[75] The effectiveness of different techniques depends on degree of obstruction, volume of sputum production, and patient cooperation. Bronchoscopy with lavage to clear secretions has been used, with clinical improvement in CF patients acutely.[76] Along with other forms of therapy in CF, there is a need for additional study regarding long-term benefits of these differing methods of secretion clearance.

Steroids

Steroids may play a role in therapy of CF patients from the standpoint of decreasing both the inflammatory response presumed to be important in mediating lung destruction and immune reactions to infection. Prolonged therapy with prednisone (2 mg/kg every other day for 4 years) in patients age 1–12 years with mild to moderate disease improved lung function and growth, and decreased the number of hospitalizations compared to a placebo-treated group without significant side effects from prednisone.[77] The stage of disease and length of therapy may affect response. For example, Pantin and colleagues treated adult CF patients with prednisone 20 to 30 mg a day for 3 weeks without significant improvement in pulmonary function, but with a possibly increased the risk of pneumonia.[78] Future studies may delineate the role of steroids in halting the progression of lung destruction.

Nutrition

Patients with CF may be malnourished for a variety of reasons, including intestinal malabsorption, increased caloric requirements with lung disease, and decreased oral intake due to lack of appetite associated with chronic illness. It is proposed that patients be placed on a high-energy balanced diet with liquid energy supplements. The improved nutritional status may result in increased respiratory muscle strength as well as improved immunity. Levy and colleagues[79] studied nutrition in 14 patients, mean age 12.9 years, who had not responded to dietary supplementation. These patients, who had oral intake during the day and nocturnal gastrostomy feeds (30% of recommended daily allowance), had subsequent increased growth and stabilization of pulmonary status compared to deterioration in matched control patients with CF. There is a suggestion that a better quality of life may result.[79] Shepherd and colleagues observed a younger age group (6 months to 11 years) who received antibiotics as needed, CPT, and diet supplementation for 6 months and demonstrated these patients' failure to thrive and frequent pulmonary infections.[42] This group was then treated with 21 days of total parenteral nutrition and demonstrated subsequent increased growth over 3–6 months and less frequent pulmonary infections in addition to improved pulmonary function. These positive results, however, may not extrapolate to an older age group.[80] The question of improved nutrition resulting in improved immune status and pulmonary function is not settled and further investigation is warranted in different age groups.

Improved nutritional status may result in increased respiratory muscle strength as well as improved immunity.

Exercise

The role of exercise in the management of CF is not well defined. Patients age 10–30 years with mild to severe disease were randomized to exercise or control groups.[81] Those in the exercise group underwent a 3-month conditioning program (running) and developed an increased exercise tolerance, decreased peak oxygen consumption, and improved spirometry and increased respiratory muscle endurance. There were no adverse side effects noted with exercise. Further long-term study is warranted, however, and caution must be used in exercising patients with borderline respiratory function, which may cause desaturation with exercise.

Other Therapy

With improvements in diagnosis of CF there have been additional efforts to find alternate therapies to prevent disease progression in CF. α_1-Antitrypsin, an elastate inhibitor, has been investigated as an option to prevent proteolytic airway damage.[82] The use of subinhibitory levels of clindamycin may be useful in the prevention of release of *Pseudomonas* elastase[83] and subinhibitory levels of aminoglycosides may be of use in inhibiting *Pseudomonas* excretion of alginate and production of siderophores.[84]

In addition to bacterial infection, viral infection has been implicated in CF deterioration.[83] Current recommendations include prevention of viral infection by immunization with measles and pertussis vaccine. The value of influenza vaccine in CF is undetermined. Amantadine and ribavirin are used with varying success. Interferon has a potential role in treatment of rhinovirus and influenza in these patients.[85]

Immunotherapy to prevent airway colonization in CF has been investigated. Polyvalent *Pseudomonas* vaccine (16 serotypes) has been used in attempts to prevent *P. aeruginosa* colonization; however, no benefit of vaccination in CF patients has been demonstrated[86] Currently, a vaccine against the three important surface components of *P. aeruginosa*, pili, liposaccharide, and alginate, is under development, which may be more effective than the polyvalent vaccine.[87]

Regulation of sodium absorption and chloride secretion, the primary defects in CF, may provide a better opportunity to improve patient outcome. Aerosolized amiloride, which blocks sodium reabsorption, reduced the viscosity of sputum, slowed progression of pulmonary deterioration, and was well tolerated.[88] More recently chloride secretion has been stimulated in nasal epithelia of patients with CF by adenosine triphosphate and uridine triphosphate, which may help reduce viscosity of secretion.[11]

Surgery and Transplantation

The role of surgery in care of the CF patient is controversial from several standpoints. Preliminary reports suggest that patients with frequent hospitalization may benefit from re-sectional surgery;[89] however, this is not the standard of care. It is recommended that resectional surgery be per-formed only after complete mapping of the bronchial tree with chest computer tomography or bronchography.[90] Management of massive hemoptysis in these patients may rarely require surgery. Additionally, surgery for long-standing atelectasis, a potential source of illness,[90] is an-other option. Lung transplantation can be performed in CF patients, however, they may be candidates for double single-lung transplantation due to problems with infection after heart-lung transplantation or scarcity of donor organs. This is discussed in greater detail in the chapter on trans-plantation.

Lung transplantation can be performed in CF patients, however they may be candidates for double single-lung transplantation due to problems with infection over heart-lung transplantation due to scarcity of donor organs.

SUMMARY

The ability to diagnose CF early in life, even antenatally, provides the opportunity for aggressive intervention early in the disease process to prevent the initial injury to the lung manifested by airway colonization and subsequent progression of the disease.

References

1. Bowman BTT, Mangos JA: Current concepts in genetics: cystic fibrosis. N Engl J Med 294:937, 1976

2. Riordan JR, Rommens JM, Kerem B et al: Identification of the cystic fibrosis genes: Cloning and characterization of complementary DNA. Science 245:1066, 1989

3. Rommens JM, Iannuzzi MC, Kerem B et al: Identification of the cystic fibrosis gene; chromo-some walking and jumping. Science 245:1059, 1989

4. Kerem B, Rommens JM, Buchanan JA et al: Identification of the cystic fibrosis gene: genetic analysis. Science 245:1073, 1989

5. Andersen DH: Cystic fibrosis of the pancreas and its relation to celiac disease. Am J Dis Child 56:344, 1938

6. The cystic fibrosis genetic analysis consortium: Worldwide survey of the ΔF508 mutation. Am J Hum Genet 47:354, 1990

7. Stuhrmann M, Macek M Jr, Reis A et al: Genotype analysis of cystic fibrosis patients in relation to pancreatic sufficiency. Lancet 335:738, 1990

8. Wood RE, Boat TF, Doerschuk CF: Cystic fibrosis. Am Rev Resir Dis 113:833, 1976

9. di Sant' Agnes PA, Davis PB: Research in cystic fibrosis. N Engl J Med 295:481, 534, 597, 1976

10. Dejonge HR: The molecular bases for chloride channel disregulation in cystic fibrosis. Acta Paediatr Scand (Suppl) 363:14, 1989

11. Knowles M, Clarke L, Boucher RC: Activation by extracellular nucleotides of chloride secretion in the airway epithelial of patients with cystic fibrosis. N Engl J Med 325:533, 1991

12. Frizzell RA, Rechkemmer G, Shoemaker RL: Altered regulation of airway epithelial cell chloride channel in cystic fibrosis. Science 233:558, 1986

13. Boucher RC, Cheng EHC, Paradiso AM et al: Chloride secretory response of cystic fibrosis human airway epithelial. J Clin Immunol 84:1424, 1989

14. Taylor CJ, Baxter PS, Hardcastle J, Hardcastle PT: Failure to induce secretion in jejunal biopsies from children with cystic fibrosis. Gut 29:957, 1988

15. Quinton PM, Bijman J: Higher bioelectric potentials due to decreased chloride absorption in the sweat glands of patients with cystic fibrosis. N Engl J Med 308:1185, 1983

16. Sato K, Sato F: Defective beta adrenergic response of cystic fibrosis sweat glands in vivo and in vitro. J Clin Invest 73:1763, 1984

17. Welsh MJ, Fick RB: Cystic fibrosis. J Clin Invest 80:1523, 1987

18. Marks MI: The pathogenesis and treatment of pulmonary infection in patients with cystic fibrosis. J Pediatr 98:173, 1981

19. Meconi AB, Pier GV, Pennington JE et al: Mucoid *Escherichia coli* in cystic fibrosis. N Engl J Med 304:1445, 1981

20. Ramphal R, Sadoff JC, Pyle M, Silipigni JD: Role of pili in the adherence of Pseudomonas aeruginosa to injured tracheal epithelium. Infect Immun 44:38, 1984

21. Hornick DB: Pulmonary host defense: defects that led to chronic inflammation of the airway. Clin Chest Med 9:669, 1988

22. Zach MS: Lung disease and cystic fibrosis—an update. Pediatr Pulmonol 8:188, 1990

23. Ramphal R, Small PM, Shands JW Jr et al: Adherence of *Pseudomonas aeruginosa* to tracheal cell injured by influenza infections or by endotracheal intubation. Infect Immun 27:614, 1980

24. Woods DE, Bass JA, Johanson JW, Strauss DC: The role of adherence in the pathogenesis of *Pseudomonas aeruginosa* lung infection in cystic fibrosis patients. Infect Immun 30:694, 1980

25. Neiderman MS, Merrill WW, Ferranti RD, Pagano KM et al: Nutritional status and bacterial binding in the lower respiratory tract in patients with chronic tracheostomy. Ann Intern Med 100:795, 1984

26. Russell NW, Gazesa P: Chemistry and biology of the alginate of mucoid strains of *Pseudomonas aeruginosa* in cystic fibrosis. Mol Aspects Med 10:1, 1988

27. Fick RB Jr, Baltimore RS, Squier SU, Reynolds HY: IgG proteolytic activity of *Pseudomonas aeruginosa* in cystic fibrosis. J Infect Dis 151:589, 1985

28. Moss RB, Hsu Y, Livingstone J: [125]-J-Clq binding and specific antibodies as indicator of pulmonary disease activity in cystic fibrosis. J Pediatr 99:215, 1981

29. Daniele RP, Henson PM, Fantone JC III et al: Immune complex injury of the lung. Am Rev Respir Dis 124:738, 1981

30. Tomashefski JF Jr, Bruce M, Goldberg HI, Dearborn DG: Regional distribution of a macroscopic lung disease in cystic fibrosis. Am Rev Respir Dis 133:535, 1986

31. Sobonya RE, Taussing LM: Quantitative aspects of lung pathology in cystic fibrosis. Am Rev Respir Dis 134:290, 1986

32. Landau LI, Phellan PD: The spectrum of cystic fibrosis. A study of pulmonary mechanics in 46 patients. Am Rev Respir Dis 108:593, 1973

33. Featherby EA, Weng TR, Crozier DN et al: Dynamics and static lung volumes, blood gas tensions, and diffusing capacity in patients with cystic fibrosis. Am Rev Respir Dis 102:737, 1970

34. Landau LI, Taussing LM, Macklem PT, Beaudry PH: Contribution of inhomogenicity of lung

units of the maximum respiratory flow–volume curve in children with asthma and cystic fibrosis. Am Rev Respir Dis 111:725, 1975

35. Darga LL, Eason LA, Zach DMS, Polgar G: Cold air provocation of airway hyperreactivity in patients with cystic fibrosis. Pediatr Pulmonol 2:82, 1986

36. Sinaasappel M: Hepatobiliary pathology in patients with cystic fibrosis. Acta Paediatr Scand (Supplement) 363:45, 1989

37. Geddes DM, Shiner R: Cystic fibrosis from lung damage to symptoms. Acad Pediatr Scand (Suppl) 363:52, 1989

38. Francis PW: Haemoglobin desaturation: its occurrence during sleep in patients with cystic fibrosis. Am J Dis Child 134:734, 1980

39. Gaskin K, Gurwitz D, Durie P et al: Improved respiratory prognosis in cystic fibrosis patients with normal fat absorption. J Pediatr 100:857, 1982

40. Kopelman H, Durie P, Gaskin K et al: Pancreatic fluid and protein hyperconcentration in cystic fibrosis. N Engl J Med 312:329, 1985

41. Boat TF: Cystic fibrosis. p. 1126. In Murray JF, Nadel JA (ds): Textbook of respiratory medicine. WB Saunders, Philadelphia, 1988

42. Gibson LE, Cooke RE: A test for concentration of electrolytes in sweat in cystic fibrosis of the pancreas utilizing pilocarpine iontophoresis. Pediatrics 23:545, 1959

43. Stern RC, Boat TF, Doershuk CF: Obstructive azoospermia as a diagnostic criterion for the cystic fibrosis syndrome. Lancet 1:1401, 1982

44. Davis PB, Del Rio S, Muntz JA et al: Sweat chloride concentrations in adults with pulmonary diseases. Am Rev Respir Dis 128:34, 1983

45. Knowles M, Gatzy J, Boucher R: Increased bioelectric potential difference across respiratory epithelia in cystic fibrosis. N Engl J Med 305:1489, 1981

46. White R, Woodward S, Leppert M et al: A closely lined genetic marker for cystic fibrosis. Nature 318:382, 1985

47. Brock DJH: Amniotic fluid alkaline phosphatase isoenzymes in early prenatal diagnosis of cystic fibrosis. Lancet 2:941, 1983

48. Hammond KB: New born screening for cystic fibrosis: results of a 2-year program in Colorado. Cystic Fibrosis Club Abstracts 25:27, 1984

49. Andersen DH: Therapy and prognosis of fibrocystic disease of the pancreas. Pediatrics 3:406, 1949

50. Boxer B: the art and science of the use of antibiotics in cystic fibrosis. Pediatr Infect Dis J 1:381, 1982

51. Marks MI: Clinical significance of *Staphylococcus aureus* in cystic fibrosis. Infection 18:53, 1990

52. Loening-Baucke VA, Mischler E, Myers MG: A placebo-controlled trial of cephalexin therapy in the ambulatory management of patients with cystic fibrosis. J Pediatr 95:630, 1979

53. Corey M, Allison L, Prober C et al: Sputum bacteriology in patients with cystic fibrosis in a Toronto hospital during 1970–1981. J Infect Dis 149:283, 1984

54. Jesnsen T, Pedersen SS, Hoiby N et al: Use of antibiotics in cystic fibrosis. The Danish approach. Antibiot Chemother 42:237, 1989

55. Wientzen R, Prestidge C, Kramer RI et al: Acute pulmonary exacerbations in cystic fibrosis: a double blind trial of tobramycin and placebo therapy. Am J Dis Child 134:1134, 1980

56. Smith AL, Redding G, Doershuk C et al: Sputum changes associated with therapy for endobronchial exacerbation in cystic fibrosis. J Pediatr 112:547, 1988

57. McLaughlin FJ, Matthew WJ Jr, Streider DJ et al: Clinical and bacteriological responses to three antibiotic regimens for acute exacerbations of cystic fibrosis: ticarcillin–tobramycin, azlocillin–tobramycin and azlocillin–placebo. J Infect Dis 147:559, 1983

58. Hodson ME, Roberts CM, Butland RJA et al: Oral ciprofloxacin compared with conventional intravenous treatment for *Pseudomonas aeruginosa* infection in adults with cystic fibrosis. Lancet 1:235, 1987

59. Szaff M, Hoiby N, Flensborg EW: Frequent antibiotic therapy improves survival of cystic fibrosis patients with chromic *Pseudomonas aeruginosa* infection. Acta Paediatr Scand 72:651, 1983

60. Grenier B: Use of the new quinolones in cystic fibrosis. Rev Infect Dis 2:S1245, 1989

61. MacLusky I, Levison H, Gold R, McLaughlin FJ: Inhaled antibiotics in cystic fibrosis: is there a therapeutic effect? J Pediatr 108:861, 1986

62. Schaad UB, Wedgwood-Krucko J, Suter S, Kraemer R: Efficacy for inhaled amikacin as adjunct to intravenous combination therapy (ceftazidime and amikacin) in cystic fibrosis. J Pediatr 111:599, 1987

63. Nathanson I, Cropp GJA, Li P et al: Effectiveness of aerosolized gentamicin in cystic fibrosis. Cystic Fibrosis Club Abstracts 26:145, 1985

64. Cooper DM, Harris M, Mitchell I: Comparison of intravenous and inhalation antibiotic therapy in acute pulmonary deterioration in cystic fibrosis. Am Rev Respir Dis 131:A242, 1985

65. Nolan G, McIvor P, Levison H et al: Antibiotic prophylaxis in cystic fibrosis; inhaled cephaloridine as an adjunct to oral cloxacillin. J Pediatr 101:626, 1982

66. Hodson ME, Penketh ARL, Batten JC: Aerosol carbenicillin and gentamicin treatment of *Pseudomonas aeruginosa* infection in patients with cystic fibrosis. Lancet 2:1137, 1981

67. Maclusky IB, Gold R, Corey M, Levison H: Long-term effects of inhaled tobramycin in patients with cystic fibrosis colonized with *Pseudomonas aeruginosa.* Pediatr Pulmonol 7:42, 1989

68. Mouton JW, Kerrebijin KF: Antibacterial therapy in cystic fibrosis. Med Clin North Am 74:837, 1990

69. Matsen JM, Bosso JA: The use fo aztreonam in the cystic fibrosis patient. Pediatr Infect Dis J 8:S117, 1989

70. Hordvik NS, Konig P, Morris D et al: A longitudinal study of bronchodilator responsiveness in cystic fibrosis. Am Rev Respir Dis 131:889, 1985

71. Wood RE, Wanner A, Hirsch J, Farrell PM: Tracheal mucociliary transport in patients with CF and its stimulation by terbutaline. Am Rev Respir Dis 111:733, 1975

72. Szach MS: Lung disease in cystic fibrosis—an updated concept. Pediatr Pulmonol 8:188, 1990

73. De Boeck C, Zinmon R: Cough versus chest physiotherapy. Am Rev Respir Dis 129:182, 1984

74. Lorin MI, Denning CR: Evaluation of postural drainage by measurement of sputum volume and consistency. Am J Phys Med Rehabil 50:215, 1971

75. Zach MS, Oberwaldner B: Chest physiotherapy—the mechanical approach to anti-infective therapy in cystic fibrosis. Infection 5:381, 1987

76. Sherman JM: Bronchial lavage in patients with cystic fibrosis: a critical review of current knowledge. Pediatr Pulmonol 2:244, 1986

77. Auerbach HS, Williams M, Kirkpatrick JA et al: Alternate day prednisone reduces morbidity and improves pulmonary function in cystic fibrosis. Lancet 2:686, 1985

78. Pantin CR, Stead RJ, Hodson ME, Batten JC: Prednisolone in the treatment of airflow obstruction in adults with cystic fibrosis. Thorax 41:34, 1986

79. Levy LD, Durie PR, Pencharz PB, Corey ML: Effects of long-term nutritional rehabilitation on body composition an clinical status in malnourished children and adolescents with cystic fibrosis. J Pediatr 107:225, 1985

80. Shepherd R, Cooksley WG, Cooke WD: Improved growth and clinical, nutritional and respiratory changes in response to nutritional therapy in cystic fibrosis. J Pediatr 97:351, 1980

81. Orenstein DM, Franklin BA, Doershuk CR et al: Exercise conditioning and cardiopulmonary fitness in CR. Chest 80:392, 1981

82. Zach MS: Pathogenesis and management of lung disease in cystic fibrosis. J R Soc Med 18:10, 1991

83. Wang EEL, Prober CG, Manson B et al: Association of respiratory viral infections with pulmonary deterioration in patients with cystic fibrosis. N Engl J Med 311:1653, 1984

84. Morris G, Brown MRW: Novel modes of action of aminoglycoside antibiotics against *Pseudomonas aeruginosa*. Lancet 1:1359, 1988

85. Stroobant J: Viral infection in cystic fibrosis. J R Soc Med 12:19, 1986

86. Langford DT, Hiller J: Prospective, controlled study of a polyvalent *Pseudomonas* vaccine in cystic fibrosis—three year result. Arch Dis Child 59:1131, 1984

87. Maguire S, Moriarty P, Tempany E, Fitzgerald M. Unusual clustering of allergic bronchopulmonary aspergillosis in children with cystic fibrosis. Pediatrics 82:835, 1988

88. Knowles MR, Church NL, Waltner WE et al: A pilot study of aerosolized amiloride for the treatment of lung disease in cystic fibrosis. N Engl J Med 322:1189, 1990

89. Schuster SR, Schwartz M, Shwachman H et al: Pulmonary surgical therapy and it long-term follow up in 52 patient with cystic fibrosis. In Sturgess JM (ed): Perspectives in cystic fibrosis: proceedings of the Eighth International Congress on Cystic Fibrosis. Imperial Press, Mississauga, Ontario, Canada, 1980

90. Fick RB, Stillwell PC: Controversies in the management of pulmonary disease due to cystic fibrosis. Chest 95:1319, 1989

AIRFLOW OBSTRUCTION DURING SLEEP

CHARLES L. BRYAN, MD
STEPHANIE M. LEVINE, MD

Sleep is normally a dynamic physiologic process that is associated with qualitative and quantitative changes in respiration tending toward hypoventilation and hypoxemia. In conditions of chronic obstructive pulmonary disease (COPD), asthma, and obstructive sleep apnea syndrome (OSAS), these changes are exaggerated, resulting in chronic hypoxemic and/or hypercapnic respiratory failure during the awake and the sleep states. This chapter examines the interrelationship between airflow obstruction and sleep. As such, it will concentrate on OSAS and COPD. It is important to understand the humoral and neurophysiologic controls placed on the different stages of sleep since specific therapeutic interventions designed to improve respiration may be successful in one stage of sleep but not in another. Therefore, the first part of this section will deal with normal changes in respiration occurring during sleep and the later sections will deal with the exaggerated malfunctions imposed by the sleep state on airflow obstruction.

Specific therapeutic interventions designed to improve respiration may be successful in one stage of sleep but not in another.

NORMAL SLEEP AND BREATHING

Sleep is divided into two physiologic subsets, nonrapid eye movement (nonREM) and rapid eye movement (REM) sleep. These two states are as different physiologically as sleep and wakefulness. NonREM sleep is further subdivided into four stages, conventionally designated as stages I, II, III, and IV. Progression through the four stages of nonREM sleep is characterized by progressive slowing of electroencephalographic activity as well as the basal metabolic rate. Therefore, stages I and II sleep are light sleeping stages and stages III and IV sleep are deep sleeping stages associated with pronounced slow wave activity on the electroencephalogram. REM sleep is a dynamic state intercalated into the nonREM stages usually after stage II. Each of these states is associated with changes in breathing.

Breathing during sleep is controlled by the same chemical

Breathing during sleep is controlled by the same chemical and mechanical feedback mechanisms that influence the brainstem during the awake state, but the response is different depending upon the stage of sleep.

and mechanical feedback mechanisms that influence the brainstem during the awake state, but the response is different depending upon the stage of sleep. During the early stages of nonREM sleep, an adult's breathing is irregular. As sleep progresses to deeper stages, breathing becomes more regular. The pattern of irregular breathing during the early stages of nonREM sleep has been compared to both Cheyne-Stokes respirations (crescendo–decrescendo tidal volumes separated by brief apneas or hypopneas) and Biot's breathing (characterized by decrescendo tidal volumes separated by brief apneas).[1] The instability of breathing during lighter stages of sleep may be attributed to two different processes.[2,3] During sleep the ventilatory response to carbon dioxide is blunted. As the carbon dioxide level rises, neurohumoral mechanisms are triggered that increase the central ventilatory drive. Minute ventilation increases, allowing carbon dioxide to be eliminated. Ultimately, there is an overshoot of this process resulting in lowering of the carbon dioxide level below threshold. Therefore, the fluxes in carbon dioxide ultimately lead to cyclic variations in ventilation. It is easy to see that patients who have a coexisting blunted carbon dioxide response in the awake state will be subject to even wider fluctuations in breathing during sleep. This condition may exist in COPD patients referred to as "blue bloaters." Another mechanism that may explain the periodic fluctuations in breathing during early stages of sleep is based on the interaction between ventilatory work and upper airway resistance. As sleep progresses, tone is lost in the upper airways, resulting in an increase in airway resistance. This change in resistance increases inspiratory work, and unless work is adequately increased to compensate, tidal volume decreases. The pathologic extreme of this process is obstructive sleep apnea, described below. Once the normal adult has progressed beyond stage II sleep, breathing becomes regular and central ventilatory drive responds to changes in carbon dioxide and oxygen similar to the awake state, although the carbon dioxide set-point is higher. The ventilation during steady nonREM sleep is lower than it is during the awake state, predominantly because of a decrease in inspiratory time relative to total ventilatory time.

Normal adult breathing during REM sleep is different. REM sleep is the stage in which dreams occur. During this stage there is an increase in central neuronal activity and a decrease in peripheral muscle activity. In general, minute ventilation becomes less dependent on intercostal muscle activity and more dependent on diaphragmatic activity. During REM sleep there are also periodic irregularities in respiration.[1,4] These irregularities are linked to episodes of rapid eye movement. When eye movements begin, there is an abrupt reduction in tidal volume followed by a more gradual increase.[5] Breathing irregularities during REM sleep are thought to be of central neuronal origin as compared to irregularities during nonREM sleep.

In summary, breathing in the normal adult is irregular initially but becomes regular as sleep deepens. REM sleep is associated with episodic rapid shallow breathing with increased dependence on diaphragmatic activity.

Breathing irregularities during REM sleep are thought to be of central neuronal origin as compared to irregularities during nonREM sleep.

Bronchial Tone and Reactivity During Sleep

Mortality in patients suffering with COPD and asthma is increased at night.[6] This realization has prompted a number of investigators to study factors affecting bronchial tone and reactivity during sleep. They have reported cyclic changes in bronchial tone. In asthmatics, these changes occur on a 24-hour cycle and are, therefore, circadian. Clark and Hetzel have shown that peak expiratory flow rate is highest in asthmatics at approximately 4:00 PM and is lowest at approximately 4:00 AM.[7] The difference in flow rate between these two time points can be as high as 50%. Bronchial tone is increased in normal subjects in the early morning hours but in them the increase is not as significant. The changes in peak expiratory flow rate appear to be related to the sleep–wake cycle. That is, asthmatics who work a night shift have their greatest increase in airway resistance upon awakening in the evening before they go to work, whereas asthmatics who work a day shift have their highest airflow resistance upon awakening in the morning.[7] Bronchial reactivity is also greatest in the early morning. This increase in bronchial reactivity is probably the sleep-time manifestation of the late asthmatic response. That is, after antigen exposure, atopic individuals turn on their bronchial inflammatory response. These changes coincide with circadian decreases in epinephrine, cAMP, and cortisol and increases in histamine.[8,9] Nocturnal increases in bronchial reactivity may also be due to esophageal reflux[10] or nocturnal airway cooling.[11]

In summary, bronchial tone increases as sleep progresses in everyone. The increase in bronchial tone does not become clinically significant, except in asthmatics. Bronchial reactivity increases as sleep progresses in susceptible atopic individuals. The resultant increase in airway resistance during inspiration will ultimately lead to decreased inspiratory flow, increased inspiratory effort, and decreased tidal volume.

OBSTRUCTIVE SLEEP APNEA SYNDROME

Any condition that increases the negativity of intraluminal airway pressure or interferes with the abductor function in the airway will predispose to the development of airway closure.

Obstructive sleep apnea syndrome (OSAS) is a multifactorial disorder that produces airway closure during sleep, resulting in hypoventilation and hypoxia. The airway closure is the result of an imbalance between the negative intraluminal airway pressure, which tends to collapse the airway, and the abductor muscles and cartilaginous support, which tend to keep the airway patent. Any condition that increases the negativity of intraluminal airway pressure or interferes with the abductor function in the airway will predispose to the development of airway closure.

Any narrowing of the upper airway lumen can be associated with increased inspiratory airway resistance. Narrowing can occur at the level of the nasopharynx, the oropharynx, or the hypopharynx. Factors affecting the patency of the upper airway can be divided into anatomic and physiologic categories (Table 1).[12]

Anatomic factors are measurable and are commonly associated with craniofacial abnormalities that can be observed on routine physical examination. Anatomic factors in OSAS subjects may reveal a posteriorly positioned maxilla and mandible, a steep occlusal plane, overerupted maxillary and mandibular teeth, proclined incisors, a steep mandibular plane, a large gonial angle, high upper and lower facial hikes, and an anterior overbite associated with a large tongue and a posteriorly placed pharyngeal wall. These abnormalities impinge on the cross-sectional area of the upper airway, subsequently leading to increased airflow resistance. Anatomic factors alone, although associated with the development of obstructive sleep apnea, are not predictive of obstructive sleep apnea.

Physiologic factors that contribute toward the development of obstructive sleep apnea include abnormalities of the pharyngeal abductor and dilator muscles, impaired recognition of increased airway resistance by the central

TABLE 1 Causes of OSAS

Anatomic	Physiologic
Macroglossia	Blunted response to carbon dioxide
Retrognathia	Blunted detection of airway resistance
Micrognathia	Loss of airway abductors
Nasal septal deviation	Alcohol
Tonsillar hypertrophy	Sedatives/hypnotics
Nasal polyps	
Pharyngeal narrowing	

nervous system, and differential recruitment of the genioglossus muscle (tongue) and the diaphragm. Numerous studies have attempted to predict the presence of obstructive apnea during sleep by examining the patient in the awake state. However, all have failed, predominantly due to two factors. The first is the failure of awake studies to predict physiologic factors affecting airway resistance during sleep. As described above, sleep is a dynamic physiologic state with different thresholds for carbon dioxide chemoreceptor sensitivity, inspiratory load resistance detection, and neurologic controls affecting tidal volume and ventilatory frequency. The second factor that has prevented the prediction of OSAS in awake-state tests involves the failure of compensatory mechanisms.

Stauffer and others measured pharyngeal cross-sectional area and pharyngeal airflow resistance in 12 overweight men with severe OSAS and normal controls.[13] They found the inspiratory airflow resistance was increased in the naso-oropharynx of patients with OSAS compared to normal control subjects but there was no difference in pharyngeal cross-sectional area while awake between the two groups. They suggested that the ability to dilate the pharynx during inspiration may be defective in patients with OSAS. Other studies have shown that the site of increased airway resistance is not necessarily associated with the specific site of airway obstruction during obstructive sleep apnea. When inspiratory airflow resistance increases, that portion of the airway soft tissue that is most pliable will be the area of collapse. In other words, the site of greatest airflow resistance may be in the nose due to septal deviation, in the nasopharynx due to polyps, at the base of the tongue due to lymphoid hyperplasia or macroglossia, or in the hypopharynx due to retrognathia or micrognathia, and the site of airway collapse in any of these conditions may be due to coaptation of the soft palate with the posterior pharyngeal wall or posterior displacement of the tongue. This difference has important implications for therapy since any procedure undertaken to decrease inspiratory airway resistance should decrease factors favoring airway collapse regardless of the actual site of airway collapse.

Other investigators have attempted to predict the presence of obstructive sleep apnea using spirometry and flow volume curves. Spirometry, including forced expiratory volume in 1 second, forced vital capacity, and maximum voluntary ventilation, are not significantly different between OSAS patients and normal subjects when matched for age and weight. Stauffer and others have shown a correlation between OSAS and expiratory/inspiratory midflow ratios and cross-sectional oropharyngeal dimensions.[14]

Some studies have shown that the site of increased airway resistance is not necessarily associated with the specific site of airway obstruction during obstructive sleep apnea.

How useful the correlation is in predicting OSAS is unknown. The expiratory flow volume loop is often abnormal in patients with variable or fixed intrathoracic or extrathoracic upper airway obstruction. This has prompted a number of investigators to evaluate the awake flow volume loop in predicting the presence of obstructive apnea during sleep.[15,16] The flow volume loop sometimes demonstrates a sawtooth pattern on the inspiratory limb that correlates with pharyngeal soft tissue vibrations during snoring. However, the flow volume loop is not consistently abnormal enough to be used as a predictive test.

Patients with OSAS have a blunted arousal response, resulting in longer hypopneas and apneas, greater oxygen desaturation, and higher CO₂.

When normal subjects experience an increase in central ventilatory drive during sleep, there is an arousal response. The increase in central ventilatory drive may be prompted by hypoxemia or increased inspiratory airway resistance. The arousal response may be represented by a true awakening or a transition from a deeper to a lighter stage of sleep. The arousal response normally becomes more blunted as sleep deepens.[17] Patients with OSAS have been shown to have a blunted arousal response, resulting in longer hypopneas and apneas, greater oxygen desaturation, and higher carbon dioxide levels. Whether this factor is a cause or result of the disorder is not clear. Failure of this compensatory mechanism is another reason why studies in awake patients are not predictive of disorders that occur during sleep.

Airway closure during sleep runs the spectrum from partial to complete obstruction. Partial obstruction occurs in nonapneic snorers. The snoring is produced by resonance of vibrating soft tissue structures in the naso-oropharynx. Partial obstruction may progress to produce a 50% reduction in tidal volume, which has been defined as "hypopnea." Recurrent hypopneas lasting over 10 seconds can also lead to nocturnal oxygen desaturation. Total cessation of airflow at the nose and mouth for over 10 seconds is defined as "apnea." During sleep muscular tone decreases according to the sleep state and the anatomic structure of the upper airways tends to collapse. When inspiratory flow resistance is increased, collapse occurs.

The prevalence of OSAS in adults is between 1 and 5% and increases with age;[18] it occurs more often in men than in premenopausal women. This difference is probably due to progesterone influences. The most common symptoms of OSAS are listed in Table 2.[19] Nocturnal symptoms include snoring, chocking or gagging, pyrosis, nocturia, and diaphoresis. The snoring varies from noisy breathing to stentorian snoring with explosive resumption of breathing. This is a complaint offered by the patient's sleeping partner and emphasizes the importance of interviewing both the

TABLE 2   Symptoms of OSAS

Nighttime	Daytime
Snoring	Sleepiness
Choking	Disorientation
Pyrosis	Decreased libido
Nocturia	Morning headaches
Diaphoresis	Fatigue
	Impaired thinking

patient and his or her partner. During the obstructive event, intra-abdominal pressure increases as a result of increased diaphragmatic activity. This may lead to acid reflux and pyrosis. Increased abdominal pressure may also cause frequent nocturia. Finally, the increase in work during obstructive apnea may produce diaphoresis.

The most common daytime symptoms associated with OSAS include excessive daytime somnolence, temporal disorientation, "sleep drunkenness," decreased libido, morning headaches, and personality changes.[20] During obstructive apnea sleep is fragmented. It is characterized by numerous arousals to lighter stages of sleep. OSAS patients have a noticeable decrease in total sleep time in nonREM sleep stages III and IV as well as in REM sleep compared to normals. Since the deeper sleep stages are responsible for the restorative function of sleep, these patients feel fatigued. This fatigue leads to hypersomnolence. OSAS patients will commonly fall asleep during repetitive or monotonous activity such as driving, eating, reading, or watching television. Therefore, driving is dangerous and the patient should be instructed not to drive until the condition is cured or controlled.

OSAS patients commonly fall asleep during repetitive or monotonous activity, such as driving, eating, reading, or watching television.

Sleep fragmentation and hypoxia lead to impaired cognitive functions.[21] Patients often awaken in the morning with disorientation and automatic behavior. For example, they will place things where they don't belong, such as placing the sugar bowl in the refrigerator. Morning headaches, which are common in patients with OSAS, may be related to vasoactive changes in cerebral blood vessels secondary to nocturnal hypoxia and/or hypercarbia. Finally, these patients exhibit personality changes consisting of emotional liability, irritability, aggressive behavior, and depression. Once the condition is properly treated, these changes resolve.

Cardiovascular Complications

During obstructive events alveolar hypoxia leads to pulmonary vasoconstriction. Since the hypoxia is global, the pul-

Chronic elevations in pulmonary arterial pressure during sleep are thought eventually to produce pulmonary hypertension in the awake state, however no prospective study has ever demonstrated this relationship.

Studies suggest a strong association between systemic essential hypertension and obstructive sleep apnea.

monary vasoconstriction is global, leading to episodic pulmonary hypertension. Chronic elevations in pulmonary arterial pressure during sleep are thought to eventually produce pulmonary hypertension in the awake state even though no prospective study has ever demonstrated this relationship. Continuous measurements of nocturnal pulmonary arterial pressures have demonstrated elevations in pulmonary arterial pressure throughout the night, with the highest readings observed in the immediate postapnea period.[22,23] These changes occur during both REM and non-REM sleep but are most prominent during REM sleep for reasons mentioned below. Patients with coexisting COPD and/or daytime hypoxemia are even more likely to develop pulmonary hypertension with sleep and sustained pulmonary hypertension during the awake state.[24]

Patients with OSAS also have been shown to have repetitive paroxysmal blood pressure elevations during sleep regardless of whether their daytime blood pressures are normal or elevated.[22] Levinson and others have demonstrated that these episodic increases in blood pressure are associated with apneic episodes.[25] In addition, Kales and others have demonstrated that OSAS was more prevalent in a population of patients with essential hypertension compared to a nonhypertensive population.[26] Finally, there is an increase in the incidence of cardiovascular deaths in patients with OSAS as well as in patients who snore.[27] These studies all suggest that there is a strong association between systemic essential hypertension and OSAS. The link between these two disorders may be associated factors such as obesity or hyperlipoproteinemias. As yet, there are no studies demonstrating a cause and effect relationship between episodic elevations of systemic arterial pressure during sleep and the development of sustained essential hypertension while awake.

Cardiac arrhythmias are also common during obstructive apneas and hypopneas. Sinus pauses may last from 2 to 13 seconds. Hemodynamically significant sinus bradycardia may occur in close to 10% of the population and paroxysmal supraventricular tachycardia and ventricular tachycardia may occur in up to 7% of the population.[28]

Diagnosis

The history is the most important screening test for OSAS. The history should be obtained from the patient as well as the patient's sleeping partner, as described above. These patients usually give a history of crescendo snoring with ventilatory pauses. They often awaken with morning headaches and cognitive impairment. The most common complaint is excessive daytime somnolence manifested as falling asleep during monotonous activities. Physical examination in these patients demonstrates that over two-thirds are overweight, ranging from mildly obese (20% over ideal body weight) to morbidly obese (more than 100% over ideal body weight). Examination of the head and neck may reveal signs associated with OSAS. Craniofacial abnormalities such as Pierre, Robin syndrome or Treacher Collins syndrome are readily apparent. Nasal polyps, retrognathia or micrognathia, tonsilar hypertrophy, nasal septal deviation, and a small oropharynx are also signs of increased airway resistance. The soft palate in habitual snorers is often erythematous and edematous and, in some patients, it may even be macerated as a result of the vibratory trauma associated with the snoring.

The definitive diagnosis of obstructive sleep apnea/sleep hypopnea syndrome rests with polysomnography. Screening tests such as pulse oximetry alone or respisomnography can be performed to separate those patients with nocturnal oxygen desaturation from normals. Since disorders other than OSAS are associated with nocturnal oxygen desaturation, particularly during REM sleep, one has to be able to link changes in oxygen saturation with changes in sleep in order to diagnose OSAS and tailor treatment specifically for a given patient. Patients with OSAS desaturate during REM and nonREM sleep, as described above, but desaturation during nonREM sleep is necessary for a diagnosis of clinically significant OSAS. Polysomnography is a test that involves measuring a number of different physiologic variables with electrodes (Table 3). The electrode signal is then amplified and recorded on paper or tape. The sleep recording is then scored for stages of sleep, apneas, and hypopneas, and changes in oxygen saturation. Extraocular movements and intercostal and anterior tibial electromyography (EMG) electrodes help separate REM from nonREM sleep. A respiratory distress index (RDI) can be generated as a threshold for the existence of OSAS. The RDI is defined as the total number of apneas and hypopneas divided by the total sleep time and multiplied by 60. Criteria for the diagnosis of OSAS are listed in Table 3. An RDI greater than 10 is usually significant. Oxygen desaturations below 90% are significant since this point is the beginning of the steep portion of the oxyhemoglobin dissociation curve. Small drops in oxygen saturation below 90% are associated with tremendous drops in arterial oxygen tension. These patients fall asleep easily and transcend into REM sleep quickly because of their sleep fragmentation. Therefore, sleep latency is usually less than 10 minutes. Sleep latency is defined as the time between bedding down and falling

Since disorders other than OSAS are associated with nocturnal oxygen desaturation, particularly during REM sleep, changes in oxygen saturation must be linked with changes in sleep to diagnose OSAS and to tailor the treatment to the patient.

TABLE 3   Standard Polysomnography Montage

Electroencephalogram
Electro-oculogram, bilateral
Submental electromyogram
Nasal/oral airflow
Electrocardiogram
Respiratory effort (pleural pressure or inductance
  plethysmography)
Oxygen saturation
Anterior tibialis electromyogram

Patients with nocturnal oxygen desaturation to less than 85% with associated nasal septal deviation, nasal polyps, or tonsilar hypertrophy require surgical correction.

asleep as determined by EEG monitoring. Early REM onset is found in many patients with OSAS, although early REM onset can also be seen in any other disorder associated with sleep fragmentation as well as with narcolepsy.

Once the diagnosis of OSAS has been established, anatomic factors contributing to increased upper airway resistance should be determined. This usually requires an otolaryngology consultation. A thorough evaluation of the nose, nasopharynx, pharynx, oropharynx, and hypopharynx should be made. Any soft tissue or bony structures encroaching on the lumen of the upper airway should be noted. Patients who demonstrate nocturnal oxygen desaturation to less than 85% with associated nasal septal deviation, nasal polyps, or tonsilar hypertrophy should be subjected to surgical correction. Treatment of patients with redundant oropharyngeal soft tissue, macroglossia, or mild retrognathia is more controversial. These patients can be further assessed with cephalometric studies. Lateral cephalometric roentgenograms are taken while the patient is sitting with eyes directed forward in a neutral head position. This projection allows a more precise measurement of structures encroaching on the airway lumen. Unfortunately, there are still no clear-cut thresholds above which surgery is clearly successful in eliminating OSAS and below which it is not. If the posterior airway space at the base of the tongue is less than 15 mm, it suggests pathologic hypopharyngeal narrowing, and surgical procedures performed above the narrowing, such as uvulopalatopharyngoplasty (UPPP), may not be successful.

Other imaging techniques include cinecomputed tomography and somnofluoroscopy. Until the diagnostic benefit of these techniques is demonstrated in clinical studies, there use should be considered mainly for research applications. Physiologic factors contributing to upper airway resistance are less easily evaluated clinically and currently are within the research arena.

Treatment

Patients with RDIs between 5 and 20, oxygen desaturation greater than 85%, and fewer than 20 apneas per hour are considered to have mild OSAS. These patients can be subjected to conservative management with diet and medication (Table 4). Patients with RDIs greater than 20, oxygen saturations below 80%, and cardiovascular complications have moderate to severe OSAS. These patients should be treated with continuous positive airway pressure (CPAP) or the surgical options detailed below.

Depression of the genioglossus muscle reflux has been noted in OSAS. Remmers and others have reported complete resolution of airway obstruction and normalization of genioglossus EMG activity after moderate weight loss.[29] The superimposition of excess weight on the abdomen and chest wall decreases lung compliance and functional residual capacity. Weight loss improves the ventilatory impairment associated with obesity.[30] Weight loss also decreases the work of breathing and improves hypoxemia due to effects on diaphragmatic motion, and decreases arterial carbon dioxide tension.

Patients with mild to moderate obesity should be placed in a supervised weight reduction program. Protriptylene is a tricyclic antidepressant drug that increases upper airway tone and decreases REM sleep. This drug has been shown to reduce nocturnal oxygen desaturation in patients with mild apnea.[31] Protriptyline and other tricyclics are associated with impotence and urinary retention, and should be considered temporary therapy while awaiting more definitive therapies such as weight loss, surgical correction, or nasal CPAP, as described below. Respiratory stimulants such as medroxyprogesterone acetate, or almitrine bismesylate are relatively contraindicated in patients with OSAS.

The use of supplemental oxygen as initial therapy for

TABLE 4 Treatment of OSAS

Conservative	Surgical
Weight loss	UPPP
Lateral position	Nasal septoplasty
Avoidance of alcohol and	Tonsilar adenoidectomy
sedatives	Mandibular osteotomy
Medication	with hyoid
Protriptyline	advancement
Oxygen	Tracheostomy
Positive airway pressure	
CPAP	
BIPAP	

The use of supplemental oxygen as initial therapy for obstructive sleep apnea is controversial. When oxygen therapy is undertaken without correcting anatomic and physiologic abnormalities, the oxygen prolongs the duration of the apnea.

Though UPPP decreases apneas and improves nocturnal oxygen saturation in many patients, it does not totally eliminate OSAS in most patients.

The treatment of choice for moderate to severe obstructive sleep apnea is inspiratory positive airway pressure support in the form of continuous positive airway pressure, inspiratory airway pressure, or variable inspiratory and expiratory positive airway pressure.

OSAS is controversial. When oxygen therapy is undertaken without correcting anatomic and physiologic abnormalities, the oxygen prolongs the duration of the apnea. This is because hypoxia in OSAS patients generates an arousal response, which is thought to be protective. Most investigators believe that supplemental oxygen should be administered to the patient whose oxygen saturation nadir remains below 85% after nasal CPAP or in whom surgery has corrected anatomic and/or physiologic factors contributing to upper airway resistance. Fletcher and others have recently reviewed the role of nocturnal oxygen therapy in patients with OSAS.[32]

Uvulopalatopharyngoplasty is a surgical procedure often performed to decrease upper airway resistance in patients with OSAS. UPPP involves resection of the uvula, distal margins of the soft palate, palatine tonsils, and any excessive lateral pharyngeal tissue. Patients with anatomic narrowing and collapse confined to the uvulopharyngeal or retropalatal region of the upper airway are considered optimal surgical candidates. Initial attempts at correcting OSAS with UPPP were successful in only 20% of patients. Recently the success rate of UPPP has increased to 66% with careful preoperative selection.[33] UPPP increases the risk of nasal regurgitation and velopharyngeal insufficiency. Currently it is indicated for patients with clinically symptomatic OSAS who have appropriate anatomic features and have not responded to more conservative measures. Even though UPPP decreases apneas and improves nocturnal oxygen saturation in many patients, it does not totally eliminate OSAS in most patients. In addition, many patients with UPPP who gain weight over time will have a resurgence of their OSAS. At worst, UPPP may allow patients to be treated with nasal CPAP who prior to the surgical procedure required prohibitive airway pressures to overcome their airway obstruction.

The treatment of choice for moderate to severe OSAS is positive airway pressure support in the form of CPAP, inspiratory positive airway pressure (IPAP), or variable inspiratory and expiratory positive airway pressure (BIPAP). Nasal CPAP acts as a pneumatic splint and decreases inspiratory airflow resistance during sleep.[34] Even though CPAP decreases inspiratory airway resistance by providing positive airflow, it actually decreases pharyngeal muscle dilator activity, but the effect is only mildly counterproductive.[34,35] Nasal CPAP is the treatment of choice for most patients with moderate to severe obstructive sleep apnea. In most cases nasal CPAP totally obliterates obstructive apneic events.[36] Nasal CPAP can be administered through a tight-fitting nasal mask or nasal pillows that are inserted directly into the nostrils. Approximately 30% of the OSAS population find nasal CPAP intolerable because of several side effects. These include rebound nasal congestion, nasal mucosal irritation, abdominal bloating, and finally, physical discomfort directly related to the fit of the device.[37] Noncompliance increases once airway pressures exceed 12 cmH$_2$O and with increasing age. Patients who are noncompliant on CPAP may find BIPAP more tolerable. BIPAP devices allow independent adjustments of inspiratory and expiratory airway pressures. Newer devices have automatic as well as demand modes and may be used actually as backup open system positive pressure ventilators. Young adult patients with OSAS may elect for UPPP or other surgical options rather than face 50–60 years of nasal CPAP use.

Other surgical procedures for the treatment of anatomic causes of OSAS include tracheostomy, mandibular osteotomy with genioglossal advancement, hyoid myotomy suspension, and bimaxillary advancement.[38] Tracheostomy is still the surgical gold standard for the treatment of moderate to severe OSAS. Tracheostomy consists of making a permanent fenestration between the tracheal lumen and the skin of the lower anterior neck. This procedure allows the free exchange of air during spontaneous breathing by bypassing any potential site of upper airway obstruction. Creation of a skin flap sewn inferiorly to the skin may be performed in order to easily locate the stoma if the tracheotomy cannula becomes dislodged.[39] A fenestrated tracheotomy tube or a tracheotomy button may be used to maintain the patency of the stoma. The tracheotomy cannula or button is plugged during the daytime to allow normal speech and ventilation. The stoma appliance remains patent at night to allow normal breathing during sleep. Tracheotomy is indicated for patients with moderate to severe obstructive sleep apnea who do not respond to more conservative measures such as nasal CPAP or UPPP. At present, other oral surgical procedures, such as mandibular advancement, are reserved for patients with retrognathia, micrognathis, or macroglossia.

All patients should be subjected to follow-up polysomnography within 6 months of therapeutic intervention for OSAS.

Tracheostomy is still the gold standard for the treatment of moderate to severe obstructive sleep apnea.

CHRONIC OBSTRUCTIVE PULMONARY DISEASE

The increase interest in OSAS over the past decade has produced renewed interest in sleep-related physiologic changes occurring in COPD patients. Often patients with

Often COPD patients who present with pulmonary hypertension or cor pulmonale out of proportion to their daytime physiologic impairment have exaggerated hypoxemia during sleep.

COPD present with pulmonary hypertension or cor pulmonale out of proportion to their daytime physiologic impairment. These patients may have exaggerated hypoxemia during sleep. In addition, sleep impacts on nocturnal breathing in various ways. Hypoxemia during sleep in COPD patients is multifactorial. Factors include hypoventilation, reductions in functional residual capacity, and changes in ventilation/perfusion matching.[40]

The major cause of hypoxemia during sleep is hypoventilation during REM sleep. As described above, breathing during REM sleep is rapid and irregular and is most severe during periods of eye movement.[41] REM sleep hypoventilation is probably due to hypotonia of the intercostal muscles and decreased activity of other accessory muscles of respiration.[42] Hypoventilation during nonREM and REM sleep also occurs due to increases in upper airway resistance. This factor probably does not significantly contribute to sleep-related hypoxemia in COPD since airway resistance is about the same during REM and nonREM sleep and most episodes of desaturation occur during REM sleep.[43] Functional residual capacity decreases during REM sleep in normal subjects.[44] This may be a contributing factor to sleep-related hypoxemia but it remains to be proven in COPD patients.

The impact of ventilation/perfusion matching on REM sleep-related hypoxemia in COPD patients has not been adequately evaluated. No techniques have been developed that allow measurement of ventilation/perfusion matching accurately in sleep COPD patients. In a group of patients with COPD, Koo and others demonstrated an average waking arterial oxygen tension drop from a mean of 62.4 ± 8.6 (SD) mmHg to a level of 48.9 ± 8.8 mmHG during sleep.[45] The carbon dioxide tension rose from a mean of 49.1 ± 5.2 mmHg to 57.4 ± 8.3 mmHg. Although the major cause of hypoxemia was hypoventilation, the alveolar-arterial oxygen differences were also increased in these patients, suggesting that ventilation/perfusion matching may also have been an important contributing factor to hypoxemia.

Cardiovascular Complications

Some investigators speculate that daytime pulmonary hypertension in COPD patients may be related to nocturnal desaturation.

As described above for OSAS, pulmonary arterial pressure increases with hypoxemia in COPD patients as well. Coccagna and others demonstrated an 18-mmHg rise in pulmonary arterial pressure when the arterial oxygen tension fell by 7 mmHg.[46] There was an associated increase in carbon dioxide tension of 7 mmHg in this study. This finding has caused some investigators to speculate that daytime pulmonary hypertension in COPD patients may be related to nocturnal desaturation. Recently, Fletcher and others compared pulmonary hemodynamics between COPD patients with nocturnal oxygen saturation and COPD patients without nocturnal oxygen desaturation. The patients with nocturnal oxygen desaturation exhibited lower resting daytime arterial oxygen tension than those who did not desaturate. They also had higher red cell masses consistent with polycythemia.[47] These findings suggest an association between daytime oxygen tensions and nighttime arterial desaturation. Which occurred first is unknown. To resolve this issue they studied an additional 13 patients matched for age, spirometric changes, daytime arterial oxygen tension, and diffusion capacity. They found that pulmonary arterial resistance was still significantly greater in patients with nocturnal oxygen desaturation than it was in patients without nocturnal oxygen desaturation. Therefore, nocturnal oxygen desaturation may be a more important determinant of pulmonary hemodynamic changes than resting daytime arterial oxygen tensions.

COPD patients also exhibit an increased incidence of atrial and ventricular arrhythmias, as described in OSAS patients. These arrhythmias tend to resolve with supplemental nocturnal oxygen therapy.[48,49]

Polycythemia is a complication of chronic hypoxia. Several investigators have attempted to determine whether daytime arterial hypoxia or nocturnal oxygen desaturation is the most important cause of polycythemia. Studies by Wedzicha and others suggest that polycythemia is more common in COPD patients with nocturnal oxygen desaturation than in patients with daytime hypoxia without nocturnal oxygen desaturation.[61] These findings need to be confirmed by additional studies.

COPD patients exhibit an increased incidence of atrial and ventricular dysrrhythmias, which tend to resolve with supplemental nocturnal oxygen therapy.

Diagnosis

Polysomnography should not be performed on all COPD patients. However, those patients presenting with polycythemia, arrhythmias, pulmonary hypertension, or cor pulmonale out of proportion to their daytime arterial oxygen tensions should be subjected to polysomnography testing to determine if they have coexisting OSAS or to determine if they have significant nocturnal oxygen desaturation during REM sleep. Otherwise, the evaluation of these patients includes routine spirometry, lung volumes, resting arterial blood gases, and diffusing capacity. Guilleminault and others have suggested that a 4% or greater drop in arterial oxygen saturation between the erect and supine position in awake COPD patients may predict profound oxygen desaturation during REM sleep.[50] This finding needs to be confirmed in additional studies.

Treatment

COPD patients who demonstrate arterial oxygen desaturation below 85% should be treated with supplemental oxygen therapy. Continuous low-flow oxygen therapy is usually prescribed in COPD patients whose daytime arterial oxygen tension is less than 55 mmHg at sea level. Therefore, many patients will require oxygen therapy without knowledge of sleep changes. Nocturnal oxygen therapy decreases nocturnal arrhythmias and sleep-related pulmonary hypertension, as described above. However, nocturnal oxygen therapy may not improve the quality of sleep.[51] The amount of oxygen required at night is usually the same as required in the daytime, that is, 1–3 L/min or the lowest amount of oxygen required to maintain arterial oxygen saturation at 90% or above. One of the hazards of oxygen therapy in COPD patients is hypercapnea. Goldstein and others demonstrated that stable COPD patients placed on nocturnal supplemental oxygen demonstrated mild increases in arterial carbon dioxide tension (less than 6 mmHg), which occurred early during the night and did not progress.[52] Therefore, nocturnal oxygen therapy is reasonably safe in COPD patients as long as they are not experiencing exacerbations. The patients who are unstable should be monitored in the hospital while initiating oxygen therapy. It is controversial whether COPD patients with isolated nocturnal oxygen desaturation and normal awake blood gases should be given supplemental oxygen.

Respiratory stimulants have also been used to improve sleep-related arterial oxygen saturation in COPD patients. Medroxyprogesterone acetate was shown to increase arterial oxygen tension by 7 mmHg and decrease arterial carbon dioxide tension by 8 mmHg during nonREM sleep in five COPD patients.[53] A subsequent study performed by Dolly and others demonstrated no benefit of medroxyprogesterone acetate in nonselected patients with COPD.[54] Almitrine bismesylate is a chemoreceptor stimulant that improves arterial oxygen tension through some unknown mechanism involving ventilation/perfusion matching. It has been used in Europe recently to improve nocturnal oxygen saturation in COPD patients.[55] Almitrine is currently not available in the United States.

ASTHMA

As described above, bronchial tone and bronchial reactivity demonstrate a circadian rhythm. The greatest increase in baseline airway resistance occurs at 4:00 AM in patients who sleep during the night. In addition, those patients with the greatest increase in baseline airway resistance during sleep have the greatest increase in bronchial activity. No one is sure why bronchial tone and reactivity increase at night in asthmatic patients. The time required for the development of these changes suggests that allergens may be involved. That is, the increase in bronchial reactivity may correspond to the late asthmatic response. Therefore, exposure to allergens before sleep will result in the release of neutrophils, eosinophils, and other mediators that potentiate bronchoconstriction.[56]

Asthmatics without chronic airflow obstruction may also exhibit mild nocturnal oxygen desaturation. These changes in nocturnal oxygen saturation have been shown to increase bronchial reactivity.[57] Whether this finding justifies nocturnal oxygen therapy in asthmatics with mild nocturnal oxygen desaturation remains to be determined. Gastroesophageal reflux may also increase bronchial reactivity during sleep, although the exact relationship between esophageal pH and bronchial reactivity is uncertain.[10] Finally, airway cooling may increase bronchial reactivity. Chen and others demonstrated that the drop in peak expiratory flow rate during sleep was attenuated in patients whose slept in a warm, humidified room.[11]

The treatment of nocturnal asthma is the same as the treatment of asthma during the awake state, with a few exceptions. Attempts should be made to neutralize gastroesophageal reflux with appropriate use of histamine blockers, antacids, and positional antireflux maneuvers. Inhaled steroids may play a prominent role in preventing a second phase response in asthmatics. Therefore, these medications should be delivered at bedtime. The inhaled steroid with the longest half-life is preferred.

Chronotherapy has received a lot of attention lately. Chronotherapy refers to the administration of medications that affect peak activity that coincides with the time of greatest clinical deterioration. For example, theophylline preparations given to patients with nocturnal asthma should have a peak effect at the time of greatest airway resistance, which is around 4:00 AM. Rhind and others have demonstrated that theophyllines disrupt normal sleep stages as defined by EEG in spite of improvements in symptoms and peak expiratory flow rates.[58] Recently, Zwillich

Chronotherapy is the administration of medications that affect peak activity that coincides with the time of greatest clinical deterioration.

and others have demonstrated that sleep quality in patients with nocturnal asthma on theophyllines was no different from sleep quality in nocturnal asthmatics who inhaled β-agonists.[59] Finally, Stewart and others have demonstrated that sustained-released terbutaline improves nocturnal airflow without impeding sleep quality in patients with nocturnal asthma.[60]

In summary, therapy in nocturnal asthmatics should be directed at attenuating increases in airway resistance during sleep. The choice of agent or agents will depend on the patient's tolerance and the drug's side effects.

References

1. Bulow K: Respiration and wakefulness in man. Acta Physiol Scand 59:1, 1963

2. Bulow KS, Engvar D: Respiration and state of wakefulness in normals, studied by spirography, capnography and EEG. Acta Physiol Scand 51:230, 1961

3. Phillipson EA: Control of breathing during sleep. Am Rev Respir Dis 118:909, 1978

4. Goodenough OR, Witkin HA, Koulach D et al: The effects of stress films on respiration and eye movement activity during REM sleep. Psychophysiology 13:313, 1975

5. Schmidt-Nowara N, Snyder MJ: A quantitative analysis of the relationship between REM and breathing in normal man. Sleep Res 12:75, 1983

6. Cochrane BM, Clark TJH: A survey of asthma mortality in patients between ages 35 and 65 in the greater London hospitals in 1971. Thorax 30:300, 1975

7. Clark TJH, Hetzel MR: Diurnal variation of asthma. Br J Dis Chest 71:87, 1977

8. Barnes P, Fitzgerald A, Brown M et al: Nocturnal asthma and changes in circulatory epinephrine, histamine and cortisol. N Engl J Med 303:263, 1980

9. Martin RJ, Cicutto LC, Ballard RD: Factors related to the nocturnal worsening of asthma. Am Rev Respir Dis 141:33–38, 1990

10. Tan WC, Martin RJ, Pandey R et al: Effects of spontaneous and simulated gastroesophageal reflux in sleeping. Am Rev Respir Dis 141(6):1394, 1990

11. Chen WY, Chai H: Airway cooling and nocturnal asthma. Chest 81:675, 1982

12. Lowe AA, Santamaria JD, Fleetham JA, Price C: Facial morphology and obstructive sleep apnea. Am J Orthod Dentofac Orthop 90:484, 1986

13. Stauffer JL, Zwillich CW, Cadieux RJ et al: Pharyngeal size and resistance in obstructive sleep apnea. Am Rev Respir Dis 136:623, 1987

14. Stauffer JL, White DP, Zwillich CW: Pulmonary function in obstructive sleep apnea. Chest 97:302, 1990

15. Hoffstein V, Wright S, Zamel N: Flow-volume curves in snoring patients with and without obstructive sleep apnea. Am Rev Respir Dis 139:957, 1989

16. Shepard JW Jr, Burger CD: Nasal and oral flow-volume loops in normal subjects and patients with obstructive sleep apnea. Am Rev Respir Dis 142:1288, 1990

17. Gugger M, Molloy J, Gould GA et al: Ventilatory and arousal responses to added inspiratory resistance during sleep. Am Rev Respir Dis 140:1301, 1989

18. Lavie P: Sleep apnea in industrial workers. p. 36. In Guilleminault C, Lugaves C (eds): Sleep/ wave disorders: natural history, epidemiology and long-term evolution. Raven Press, New York, 1983

19. Stoohs R, Guilleminault C: Obstructive sleep apnea syndrome or abnormal upper airway resistance during sleep. J Clin Neurophysiol 7:83, 1990

20. Hudgel DW: Neuropsychiatric manifestations of obstructive sleep apnea: a review. Int J Psychiatr Med 19(1):11, 1989

21. Finley LJ, Bowden JT, Powers JC et al: Cognitive impairments in patients with obstructive sleep apnea associated hypoxemia. Chest 90:686, 1986

22. Tilkian AG, Guilleminault C, Schroeder JS et al: Hemodynamics in sleep-induced apnea studies during wakefulness and sleep. Ann Intern Med 85:714, 1976

23. Shepard JW: Gas exchange and hemodynamics during sleep. Med Clin North Am 69:1243, 1985

24. Fletcher EC, Schaaf JM, Miller J, Fletcher JG: Long-term cardiopulmonary sequelae in patients with sleep apnea and chronic lung disease. Am Rev Respir Dis 135:525, 1987

25. Levinson PD, Millman RP: Causes and consequences of blood pressure alterations in obstructive sleep apnea. Arch Intern Med 151:455, 1991

26. Kales A, Cadieux RJ, Shaw LC et al: Sleep apnea in a hypertensive population. Lancet 2:1005, 1984

27. Waller PC, Bhopas RS: Is snoring a cause of vascular disease? an epidemiologic review. Lancet 1:143, 1989

28. Guilleminault C, Connolly S, Winkle R: Cardiac arrhythmia during sleep in 400 patients with sleep apnea syndrome. Am J Cardiol 52:490, 1983

29. Renners JE, DeGroot WJ, Sauerland EK: Neural and mechanical factors controlling pharyngeal occlusion during sleep. p. 40. In Guillemault C, DeMent W (eds): Sleep apnea syndromes. Allen R. Liss, New York, 1978

30. Luce JM: Respiratory complications of obesity. Chest 78:626, 1980

31. Smith PL, Haponik EF, Allen RP, Bleecher ER: The effects of protriptyline in sleep-disordered breathing. Am Rev Respir Dis 127:8, 1983

32. Fletcher EC, Munafo DA: role of nocturnal oxygen therapy in obstructive sleep apnea. When should it be used? Chest 98:1497, 1990

33. Shepard JW Jr, Olsen KD: Uvulopalatopharyngoplasty for treatment of obstructive sleep apnea. Mayo Clin Proc 65:1260, 1990

34. Strohl KP, Redline S: Nasal CPAP therapy, upper airway muscle activation and obstructive sleep apnea. Am Rev Respir Dis 134:555, 1986

35. Sullivan CE, Issa FG, Berthon-Jones M et al: Reversal of obstructive sleep apnea by continuous positive airway pressure applied through the nares. Lancet 2:862, 1981

36. Stohes-Dickens A, Jenkins NA, Chambers GW: CPAP use. Sleep Res 18:223, 1989

37. Sanders MH, Gruendl CA, Rogers RM: Patient compliance with nasal CPAP therapy for sleep apnea. Chest 90:330, 1986

38. Riley R, Powell N, Guilleminault C: Inferior osteotomy of the mandible and hyoid myotomy suspension: a new procedure for obstructive sleep apnea. Otolaryngol Head Neck Surg 94:589, 1986

39. Koopmann CF Jr, Moran WB Jr: Surgical management of obstructive sleep apnea. Otolaryngol Clin North Am 23:787, 1990

40. Douglas NJ: Are sleep studies necessary in COPD? Am Rev Respir Dis. Suppl:943, 1990

41. Gould GA, Gugger M, Molloy J et al: Breathing pattern and eye movement density during REM sleep in man. Am Rev Respir Dis 138:874, 1988

42. Johnson MW, Remmers JE: Accessory muscle activity during sleep in chronic obstructive pulmonary disease. J Appl Physiol 57:1011, 1984

43. Lopes JM, Tabachnik E, Muller NL, Levison H, Bryan AC: Total airway resistance and respiratory muscle activity during sleep. J Appl Physiol 54:773, 1983

44. Hudgel DW, Martin RJ, Johnson B, Hill P: Mechanics of the respiratory system and breathing pattern during sleep in normal humans. J Appl Physiol 56:133, 1984

45. Koo KW, Sax DS, Snider GL: Arterial blood gases and pH during sleep in chronic obstructive pulmonary disease. Am J Med 58:663, 1975

46. Coccagna G, Lugaresi E: Arterial blood gases and pulmonary and systemic arterial pressure during sleep in chronic obstructive pulmonary disease. Sleep 1:117, 1978

47. Fletcher EC, Luckett RA, Miller T et al: Pulmonary vascular hemodynamics in chronic lung disease patients with and without oxyhemoglobin desaturation during sleep. Chest 95:757, 1989

48. Tirlapur VG, Mir MA: Nocturnal hypoxemia and associated electrocardiographic changes in patients with chronic obstructive airway disease. N Engl J Med 306:125, 1982

49. Shepard JW, Garrison MW, Grither DA et al: Relationship of ventricular ectopy to nocturnal oxygen desaturation in patients with chronic obstructive pulmonary disease. Am J Med 78:28, 1985

50. Guilleminault C, Cumminshey J, Motta J: Chronic obstructive airflow disease and sleep studies. Am Rev Respir Dis 122:397, 1980

51. Calverley PMA, Brezinova V, Douglas NJ et al: The effect of oxygenation on sleep quality in chronic bronchitis and emphysema. Am Rev Respir Dis 126:206, 1982

52. Goldstein RS, Romaharan V, Bowes G et al: Effect of supplemental nocturnal oxygen on gas exchange in patients with severe obstructive lung disease. N Engl J Med 310:425, 1984

53. Skatrud JB, Dempsey JA, Iber C, Berssenbrugge A: Correction of CO_2 retention during sleep in patients with chronic obstructive pulmonary diseases. Am Rev Respir Dis 124:260, 1981

54. Dolly FR, Block AJ: Medroxyprogesterone acetate and COPD effect on breathing and oxygenation in sleeping and awake patients. Chest 83:469, 1983

55. Connaughton JJ, Douglas NJ, Morgan AD et al: Almitrine improves oxygenation when both awake and asleep in patients with hypoxia and carbon dioxide retention caused by chronic bronchitis and emphysema. Am Rev Resir Dis 132:206, 1985

56. Mohiuddin AA, Martin RJ: Circadian basis of the last asthmatic response. Am Rev Respir Dis 142(5):1153, 1990

57. Denjeau A, Roux C, Herve P et al: Mild isocapnic hypoxia enhances the bronchial response to methacholine in asthmatic subjects. Am Rev Respir Dis 138:789, 1988

58. Connaughton JJ, McFie J, Douglas NJ, Flenley DC: Sustained release choline theophyllinate in nocturnal asthma. Br Med J 291:1605, 1985

59. Zwillich CW, Naegley SR, Ciccuto L et al: Nocturnal asthma therapy inhaled by bitolterol versus sustained raised theophylline. Am Rev Respir Dis 139:470, 1989

60. Stewart IC, Rhind GB, Power JT et al: Effects of sustained release terbutaline on symptoms and sleep quality in patients with nocturnal asthma. Thorax 42:797, 1987

61. Wedzicna JA, Cotes PM, Empey DW et al: Serum immunoreactive erythropoietin and hypoxic lung disease with and without polyeythemia. Clin Sci 69:413, 1985

INDEX

Page numbers followed by the letter *f* refer to figures; those followed by *t* refer to tables.